the **everything you need to know** about **diabetes cookbook**

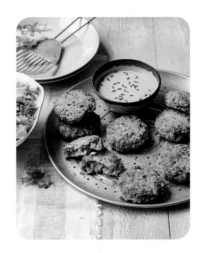

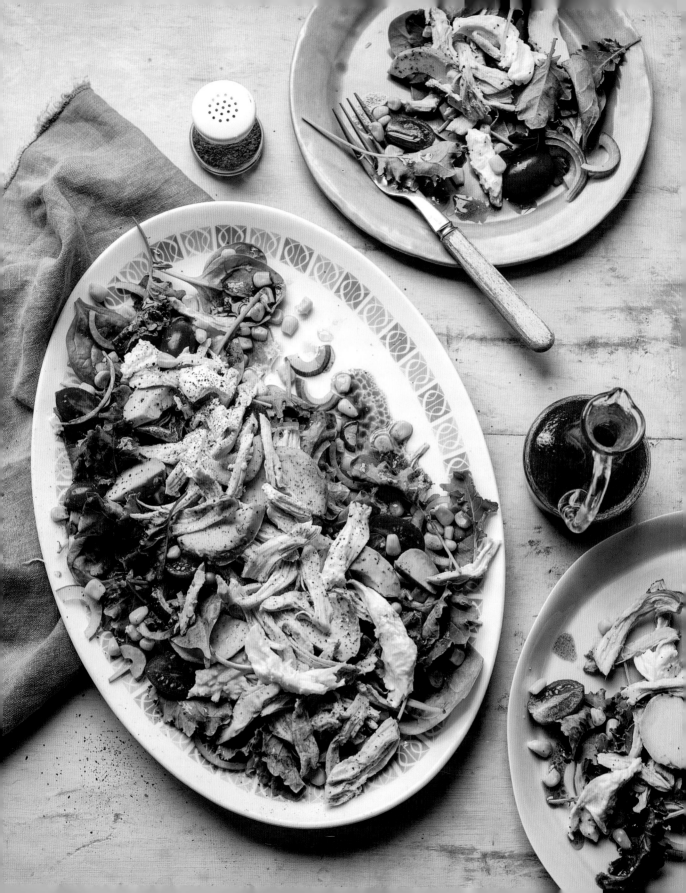

the **everything you need to know** about **diabetes cookbook**

expert advice, plus 70 recipes complete with nutritional breakdowns

Dr Karin M Hehenberger, MD, PhD

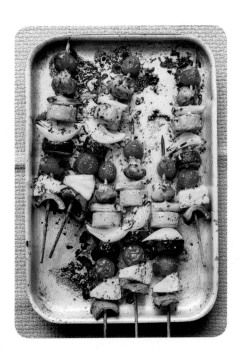

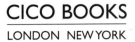

CICO BOOKS
LONDON NEW YORK

This book is dedicated to my parents who gave me life, and who continually and heroically fight with and for me to keep it.

Published in 2017 by CICO Books
An imprint of Ryland Peters & Small Ltd
20–21 Jockey's Fields   341 E 116th St
London WC1R 4BW   New York, NY 10029
www.rylandpeters.com

10 9 8 7 6 5 4 3 2 1

A CIP catalog record for this book is available from
the Library of Congress and the British Library.

ISBN: 978-1-78249-435-5

Printed in China

Part 1 and the Conclusion were previously
published through Lulu.com as *Ten Things You
Need to Know About Living with Diabetes* by
Dr Karin M Hehenberger.

Editor: Clare Churly
Photographer: Ria Osborne
Home economist: Sue Henderson
Food stylist: Luis Peral

Commissioning editor: Kristine Pidkameny
Senior editor: Carmel Edmonds
Art director: Sally Powell
Production controller: David Hearn
Publishing manager: Penny Craig
Publisher: Cindy Richards

Notes to read before you start cooking

• Both American (US cups/imperial) and British (metric) measurements and ingredients are included in these recipes for your convenience. However, it is important to work with one set of measurements and not alternate between the two within a recipe.

• Eggs are US large and UK medium unless stated otherwise.

Important note

The views expressed in this book are those of the author and readers are urged to consult a relevant and qualified medical practitioner from their diabetes care team for individual advice before beginning any dietary regime. While every attempt has been made to ensure the medical information in this book is correct and up to date at the time of publication, the Publishers accept no responsibility for consequences of inappropriate use of any dietary regime.

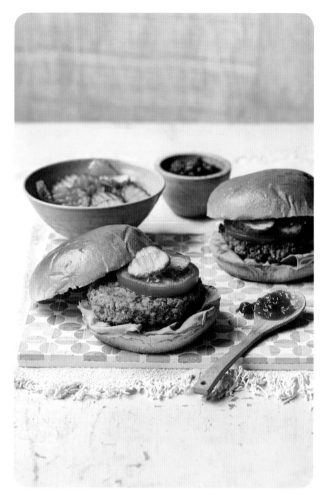

Contents

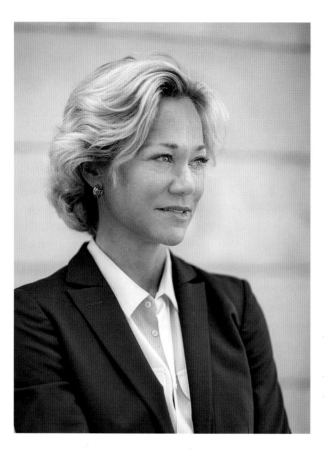

Introduction

As both a medical doctor and a person with diabetes, I know how difficult it is to accept your diagnosis and to adjust your lifestyle to deal with a chronic condition, such as diabetes. In this book you will find the top things I think you ought to know as a person with diabetes or as a person who loves and cares about someone with diabetes.

I received a diagnosis of type 1 diabetes as a teenager living in Sweden, and it affected my career choices and my life in a dramatic way. I decided early on to learn as much as possible about my disease and figure out a way to beat it, but I never accepted the disease as a part of me. My journey with diabetes taught me to face adversity with good humor and to never, ever give up. However, it also affected my confidence, love for life, and belief in my future. For a long period of time, I lived in the moment and did not expect to be around for many years. I have studied diabetes from more angles than most, first submerging myself into medical science as a scientist and clinician, and later as an analyst of companies and developer of drugs and devices. I have learned that sharing our stories, struggles, and victories may be the best way to overcome issues related to the disease and to live a life beyond survival mode.

In the first part of this book, I describe issues, situations, and problems that are part and parcel of daily life with diabetes, and are sometimes things you would have never considered prior to being diagnosed. For each one, I give you advice and tips on how to deal with them, and share my personal experience of them. In Part 2, I explain the benefits of a healthy, nutritionally balanced diet (which is good for everyone, not just those with diabetes), and how to approach adjusting your diet accordingly. There is also a collection of recipes for breakfast, light meals and salads, main meals, sides and dips, and desserts and treats. All have been designed to work with a diabetic diet and are recipes I would personally eat and enjoy.

My journey has now reached a stage where I am more comfortable with my condition. It has taken twenty-five years of living with type 1 diabetes, going through brutal complications, fighting fear and pain, and ending up with one of my father's kidneys and the pancreas of a young deceased donor. My father's sacrifice and the generosity of the family who donated their daughter's organs saved my life and made it worth living. I will be forever grateful, and I want to spend the rest of my life doing good for others while still doing well for my family and myself.

I hope that by reading this book you will learn some new facts, but that you will also better understand how to address your condition and discover fresh ways of living practically.

Above all, stay positive, be active, remain open to new ideas, and never hesitate to reach out to others for help and advice!

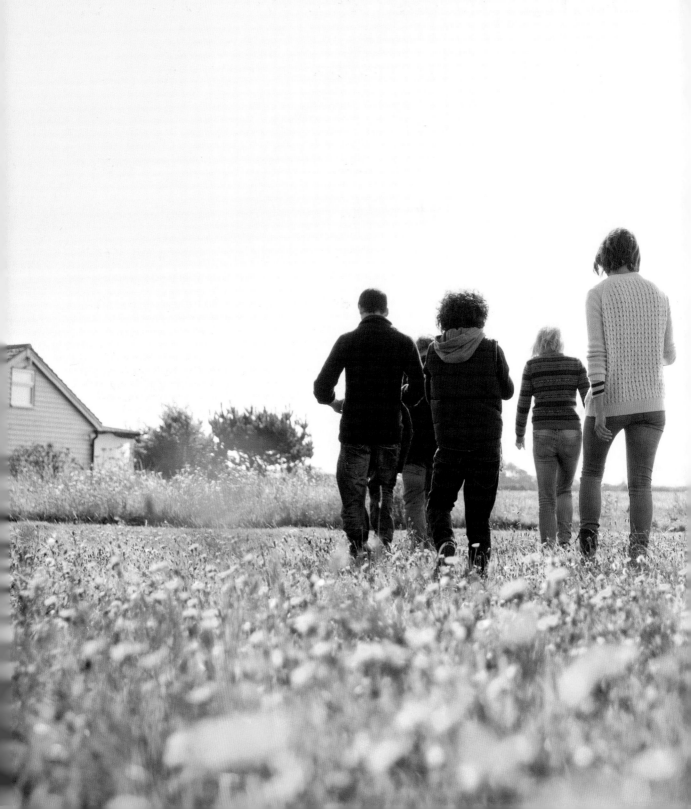

PART 1: Living Well with Diabetes

1 Being Diagnosed with Diabetes

To receive a diagnosis that you have a chronic disease is a daunting experience, since the very word "chronic" implies that it will never go away. In contrast to the flu, a urinary infection, or even certain kinds of cancer, type 1 diabetes (T1D) does not have a cure yet, although billions of dollars have been invested in the research and development of new technologies and therapeutic drugs intended to treat the disease.

T1D and T2D

There are two major types of diabetes: type 1 (T1D) and type 2 (T2D). Both diseases require diet and behavior modification as part of their treatment and may lead to serious complications, such as heart, eye, nerve, and kidney disease in the long term and loss of consciousness in the short term.

T1D is an autoimmune disease that requires lifelong treatment with insulin for survival. Autoimmune means that the body's own immune system targets the healthy cells in the body instead of fighting outside threats, such as bacteria or a virus. Examples of other autoimmune diseases are multiple sclerosis and celiac disease. T1D is generally diagnosed in children, adolescents, and young adults. About 200,000 Americans under the age of twenty are estimated to have diabetes (Centers for Disease Control and Prevention—CDC) and in 2008 and 2009, almost 20,000 young people were diagnosed with T1D and 5,000 were diagnosed with T2D each year. In the UK, there are about 31,500 children and young people under the age of nineteen with diabetes, and the vast majority of them have T1D (*Diabetes Facts and Stats: 2015*).

Scientists still don't know exactly what causes diabetes. There is clearly a genetic component since people with T1D have a higher risk of having children with the disease. But interestingly, only 10 percent of people with T1D have a relative with diabetes. In my case, I was the first one in my family who developed this disease.

There is also an environmental component to T1D, and since the highest incidence in the world is in Scandinavia, where I am from, a great deal of research has been conducted into the food, environment, and even the greatly increased exposure of young children to vaccines and antibiotics in that area of the world. The "hygiene hypothesis"—that children are being exposed to fewer infections, in part because of clean water supplies, uncontaminated food and milk, improved sanitation, and higher standards of cleanliness—may be related to all autoimmune diseases. In countries where hygiene is poor, there appears to be a low incidence of all autoimmune diseases, including T1D.

Some speculate that T1D is triggered by infection, which somehow overstresses the pancreas. As a result, the immune system mistakenly targets the pancreas, instead of the

DIABETES FACTS AND FIGURES

- According to the Centers for Disease Control and Prevention (CDC), 29.1 million Americans had diabetes in 2012 (*National Diabetes Statistical Report*, 2014)—this means that almost 10 percent of all Americans have some form of the disease—and the number of new cases of diabetes per year is increasing faster than the population grows

- From 2001 to 2009 in America, T1D among youth increased 23 percent and T2D among youth increased 21 percent (Mayer-Davis et al., 2012; Dabelera, D. et al., 2012)

- According to Diabetes UK, it is estimated that 3.5 million people have been diagnosed with diabetes in the UK (*Diabetes Facts and Stats: 2015*) and it is predicted 549,000 have diabetes that is yet to be diagnosed: this means that over 4 million people are estimated to be living with diabetes in the UK at present, which represents 6 percent of the UK population or 1 in every 16 people having diabetes (diagnosed and undiagnosed)

- Epidemiologists estimate that by 2030, 550 million people will have diabetes worldwide (International Diabetes Federation)—of these, 183 million will be unaware of their condition

- In the US only, one in three people may have diabetes by 2050 (CDC)

- Diabetes requires much medical care, so the financial burden on society due to diabetes is great, with total costs approaching $250 billion in 2012 (CDC)

- Diabetes was the underlying cause of death of almost 70,000 Americans in 2012 and a contributor to more than an additional 230,000 deaths, making it the seventh most deadly disease (CDC)

- People with diabetes are two to four times more likely than other people to die of heart disease, and diabetes is also the leading cause of kidney failure, accounting for 44 percent of all new cases, as well as the leading cause of new cases of blindness in adults (CDC, 2012)

Karin's story: ACCEPTING MY DIAGNOSIS

On July 5, 1989, two days before my seventeenth birthday, I received a diagnosis of T1D. It was the worst day of my life up to that point, and to this day, it still is. I felt as if I had become an entirely different person, one with a chronic disease who had lost in life. I had been a member of the Swedish National Junior Tennis Team. I ran and I skied. I was competitive about everything, even crossing the street; I wanted to get to the other side first. I never questioned my ability to win or my ability to control my body.

I was not only an athlete. My parents placed a high priority on academic achievement. My father is a quantum chemist, and my mother a highly educated stay-at-home mom. I worked hard and did well in school. In particular I excelled at the sciences and had already developed what would become a lifelong fascination with medicine.

That summer, I played in a major tennis tournament in southern Sweden. I was playing hard every day and had reached the finals, but I was also experiencing the first symptoms of diabetes. No one in my family had ever received a diagnosis of diabetes, and my parents and I did not recognize any of the signs.

I was drinking enormous amounts of fluids, which ran right through me so that I was constantly peeing. I was losing weight daily, which didn't bother me since I thought it made me look better (I was a typical teenage girl). But I was getting weaker, too, and developing cramps in my lower legs. My vision became blurry; I was always a little nauseated and lost all interest in food. After the tournament, I went to my grandparents' country home in northern Sweden to rest. It was they who finally recognized that what I was experiencing were symptoms of diabetes and took me to the hospital. There, blood tests revealed that my blood sugar level was sky high; I had T1D.

"Seventy years ago, you would have been dead," the nurse told me.

Her comment was the first of many that made me feel different and vulnerable. I was no longer a strong young woman, but someone who would die if she didn't have access to insulin injections. Indeed, fear crept into my everyday life, and many nights I had a nightmare about not being allowed onto Noah's Ark. Like most teenagers, I struggled with fitting in with my peers, and getting a diagnosis of a life-threatening and debilitating disease made doing so much more difficult.

No one in my family had ever received
a diagnosis of diabetes, and my parents
and I did not recognize the signs

bacteria or virus causing the infection. I, for example, had three serious bouts of tonsillitis, all requiring treatment with antibiotics, in the spring before I got a diagnosis of diabetes. Were those infections related to my condition? Not enough is known yet to say for sure. Fortunately, much is known about how to deal with the disease once it is diagnosed.

T2D is all too common in the Western world, accounting for 90 to 95 percent of the total 29.1 million cases, with T1D being responsible for the remaining 5 to 10 percent. Another 86 million have prediabetes—blood glucose levels higher than normal, but not yet in the diabetic range. Thirty percent of people with prediabetes develop full-blown T2D. T2D is also believed to have a genetic component; people who are genetically predisposed to obesity are more likely to develop the disease. For example, when one identical twin develops T2D, the chances of the other twin developing it are 80 percent, whereas in T1D, the risk is less than 50 percent.

The reason T2D is often considered a "disease of the Western world" is because it mainly affects those who are overweight, eat poorly, are not sufficiently active, and make other lifestyle choices that are detrimental to their health. In the United States it has reached almost epidemic proportions. It tends to affect people later in life, at middle age or older. Unfortunately, that is changing because obesity is increasing, largely as a result of our unhealthy Western lifestyle. Now even children are developing T2D, which means that millions of young adults are facing (and will face) the late-stage complications of the disease.

Both T1D and T2D are chronic diseases and are diagnosed based on blood glucose levels as indicated by the following criteria:

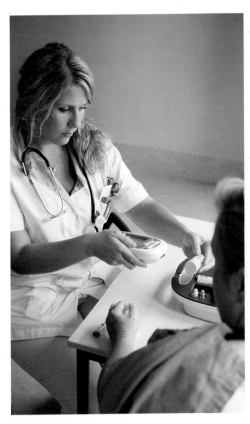

- a blood glucose level of 126 milligrams per deciliter (mg/dL) or higher after an eight-hour fast as measured by the fasting glucose test;

- a blood glucose level of 200 mg/dL or higher two hours after drinking a beverage containing 75 grams of glucose dissolved in water as measured by the oral glucose tolerance test;

- a random blood glucose level of 200 mg/dL or higher, along with the presence of diabetes symptoms;

- an HbA1c level of 6.5 percent or higher—the long-term measurement for glucose that measures the percentage of red blood cells that are glycosylated (red blood cells in which the hemoglobin is bound to glucose).

People with T1D or T2D are unable to control glucose levels in their blood due to an inability to manufacture a sufficient amount of insulin. That means, if unregulated, the dangerously elevated amount of sugar in their bloodstream adversely affects organs, vessels, and tissues. If people with diabetes do not take proper care of themselves, the long-term complications are the same for both types of diabetes: eye, kidney, and nerve disease, as well as cardiovascular complications.

Ketoacidosis and hyperglycemia

Based on how the disease is diagnosed, its causes, and, importantly, my own reaction and experiences, I want to help families and individuals with the disease deal with the situation.

Because the incidence of diabetes is growing to almost epidemic proportions, it is important that people—particularly the family and friends of people with diabetes—be educated about the symptoms of ketoacidosis and hyperglycemic coma in the case of T1D, and the warning signs before diagnosis in the case of T2D. Ketoacidosis is a metabolic state associated with high concentrations of ketone bodies formed by the breakdown of fatty acids and the deamination of amino acids—i.e. what happens when the body breaks down fat for energy. The two common ketones produced in humans are acetoacetic acid and beta-hydroxybutyrate.

Ketoacidosis is a dangerous, pathological metabolic state marked by extreme and uncontrolled ketosis (when you have hyperglycemia—high blood sugars—and your body uses ketones instead of glucose as energy, which is extremely dangerous). In ketoacidosis, the body fails to adequately regulate ketone production, causing such a severe accumulation of keto acids that the pH of the blood is substantially decreased (acidosis). In extreme cases ketoacidosis can be fatal.

Ketoacidosis is common in untreated T1D and is usually accompanied by insulin deficiency, hyperglycemia, and dehydration. The lack of insulin in the bloodstream prevents glucose absorption and can cause unchecked ketone body production (through fatty acid metabolism) potentially leading to dangerous glucose and ketone levels in the blood. Hyperglycemia results in glucose overloading the kidneys and spilling into the urine. Dehydration results from the osmotic movement of water into urine, exacerbating the acidosis. Ketoacidosis can be smelled on a person's breath, due to acetone (a type of ketone body), often described as smelling like fruit.

Recognizing symptoms

A child who experiences increased fatigue, frequent urination, excessive thirst, and weight loss should be seen by a doctor immediately. Intervention at this point could prevent hospitalization upon diagnosis and might avert some of the damage that occurs before diagnosis and before the child's blood sugar indicates that he or she has full-blown

A child who experiences increased fatigue, frequent urination, excessive thirst, and weight loss should be seen by a doctor immediately— early intervention can prevent hospitalization

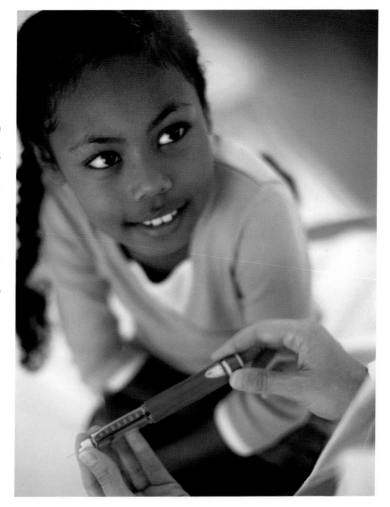

diabetes. Beta cells in the pancreas secrete insulin, and during the critical stage prior to clinical diagnosis there may be ways in the future to protect those cells from damage and thus allow for delayed diagnosis or a milder disease.

In adults, the symptoms of T2D are much more subtle and can go unnoticed for years. There is no reason for people not to have annual physical exams and blood work done, including glucose tests. If you are overweight—even slightly—you should have blood work and blood pressure tests performed more frequently. Today, pharmacies and mini-clinics are excellent options for this kind of testing, simplifying the process for everyone and reducing the cost and time required.

Once you have received your diagnosis, doctors, nurses, and other health care professionals will explain how the condition should be managed and how it will affect your life. This information can be difficult to take in. When you first get your diagnosis,

I recommend having a family member or friend accompany you when the doctors explain the new life you are required to lead. They can listen, maybe ask some questions, and take notes, but perhaps most importantly, they can be there for you and hold your hand, both literally and figuratively. This will not be the only conversation you have with your doctor and other medical professionals about the topic, so try to take in what you can but do not worry if you need to go over the information more than once.

The practical aspects of dosing insulin, counting carbohydrates, and pricking your fingers for blood glucose values multiple times a day can be overwhelming. I found, however, that the serious health consequences of *not* perfectly managing the disease scared me much more, and I really did not want to hear about them. You can't ignore the fact that your life has changed. Adjusting to being dependent on a drug such as insulin and realizing you have to modify your lifestyle can be difficult. Indeed, some people will be in denial about the seriousness of their condition. It is important to understand that only you can manage your disease, and that by doing so with medicines, diet, and exercise, you can have a long, healthy, and enjoyable life.

! REMEMBER

- Type 1 (T1D) and type 2 (T2D) diabetes are both diagnosed by determining your blood glucose level.

- T1D is an autoimmune disease usually diagnosed in children, adolescents, and young adults.

- T2D is most often triggered by lifestyle factors, including being overweight, lack of exercise, and an unhealthy diet.

- Receiving a diagnosis of diabetes can be a shock and can affect your ability to absorb and process information. Bring a close friend or family member with you to doctors' appointments, not just for emotional support, but to take notes and ask questions that may not occur to you.

- It is your responsibility to manage your disease, but if you do so, you can live a long and healthy life.

2 Your Diabetes Team

After you have received your diagnosis, you, along with your doctor and other health care professionals, will need to create the best possible treatment program for you—and not just from a medical perspective. The reality is that people with diabetes require many touchpoints within the health care system.

Primary care

If you have T1D, your basic medical care, which includes monitoring and managing your blood sugar levels, will be handled by an endocrinologist or a doctor who specializes in treating diabetes. (Unfortunately, there are not enough of these doctors in the United States to handle the more than 100 million people at risk or with a diagnosis.) If you have T2D, you may be treated by a primary care doctor, who may or may not be knowledgeable about treating and managing diabetes. It is important to interview your doctor and not settle on one until you find someone who has sufficient experience with and knowledge of all the intricacies of your condition.

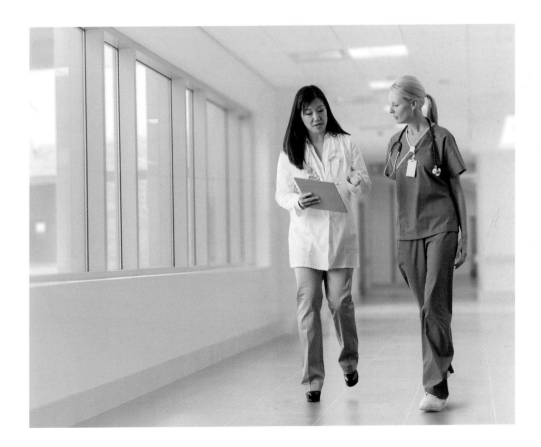

Managing diabetes is not just about controlling your blood sugar levels; your primary care doctor must function as a coordinator for your entire health care team. This team should include a nurse who can help manage your blood sugar levels, respond to daily requests, and talk to you about technical problems with devices or drugs. The nurse often has more practical skills than the doctor; for example, if you have a blood glucose meter, the nurse can help you download glucose values from the meter through a cable or even wirelessly to the nurse's or doctor's computer to help manage dosing, carbohydrate loads, exercise, etc.

Diet and fitness

Another important member of the team is the dietician. Your blood sugar levels are affected by the food you eat in a major way; knowing what foods can help you manage the disease and which ones to avoid will be essential. You will also need a fitness professional or coach to help you design a good exercise program. Your primary care doctor may have a recommendation, or you may be able to get help from a local gym, YMCA, or community center. The way you exercise when injecting insulin is different from when you don't, and it is very beneficial to understand what each situation requires.

Additional specialists

Unfortunately, diabetes involves the risk of damage to the small (micro) and large (macro) blood vessels (vasculature). This is very common in people with T2D who may have had the disease for years before getting a diagnosis and often have some complications already. For this reason, it is critical to be seen by a retinal specialist. This doctor examines you to determine whether you have diabetic retinopathy, a condition affecting the blood vessels in the back of the eye that may lead to blindness if untreated. In fact, the CDC notes that diabetes is the leading cause of blindness in people younger than sixty-five in the Western world. The other key player on your team is the nephrologist, or kidney doctor. Similar to the eyes, the kidneys have many small blood vessels that may be damaged by longstanding diabetes. In fact, a person who has had diabetes for more than ten years likely has some signs of kidney disease; however, in most cases it will not progress if blood pressure and blood sugar levels are closely managed.

A cardiologist should be part of the team as well, particularly if you have received a diagnosis of T2D and are older than fifty. Annual exams are crucial. The World Heart Federation says diabetes increases the risk of heart disease by two to four times, and in women that number may be even higher.

A foot doctor or podiatrist is another component of the diabetes team. The extremities, especially your feet, are vulnerable to blood sugar fluctuations, as well as poor circulation and nerve damage. The latter can cause loss of sensitivity, and all three can lead to poorly healing wounds, followed by amputations in the worst cases. Your dental health may also be affected by diabetes, so identifying a good dentist, and possibly an orthodontist, is very important too. Last, your team must include psychological and social support. It isn't easy to live with a chronic disease. You have to manage multiple doctors' visits, as well as deal with devices and drugs on a daily basis. Everyone needs someone to talk to, and having an impartial ear can alleviate the feeling of being dependent on or a burden to your family and loved ones. A social worker or health advocate can help with insurance issues and provide information about benefits. It is very costly to have diabetes, and there are many resources available of which you may not be aware.

It is important that people with diabetes get access to proper care in order to prevent the serious complications associated with the disease. The consequences of poor management are grave, both medically and economically, and the entire health care system should be very active in prevention. This can happen through a greater effort to educate people with diabetes about their condition, providing less expensive alternatives to junk food, and emphasizing exercise and healthful living in young people through school programs.

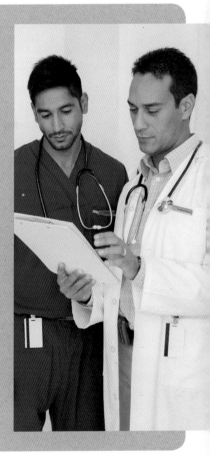

! REMEMBER

- You need a team to help you manage your diabetes.

- Your key team member will be your primary care doctor, endocrinologist, or diabetes specialist.

- Your team should include a nurse in your doctor's office, dietician, fitness professional, retinal specialist, nephrologist, cardiologist, podiatrist, dentist and possibly an orthodontist, counselor, and social worker or health advocate.

- Preventive efforts are critical in diabetes management to avoid medical and economic consequences for the individual and society.

3 | Going Low

For people living with diabetes, sugar is not only something we consider when we eat, but something we measure in our blood several times a day. Blood glucose levels determine our mood and energy in the short term, and if our blood glucose is unstable, it can lead to serious long-term consequences for our health.

In diabetes terms, "going low" or, in more technical terms, being hypoglycemic, is a very specific concept, defined by a blood sugar level that is less than 70 mg/dL. However, it is important to realize that different people have different tolerances for low blood sugar levels, and some people, especially those with longstanding diabetes, may suffer from hypo-unawareness. In other words, despite having dangerously low blood sugar, they do not exhibit the normal symptoms of low blood sugar, so it is much harder for those around them to intervene.

Going low is a scary event for someone with diabetes. We all know that when we skip a meal or exercise too hard without having consumed enough calories to support the expenditure of energy, we may feel shaky, develop a headache, and/or become irritable. For someone with diabetes, these feelings are even more intense. Eventually, the person will lose consciousness, and without intervention, he or she could die. Every year, one out of every twenty people with T1D dies from hypoglycemia; this occurs more commonly

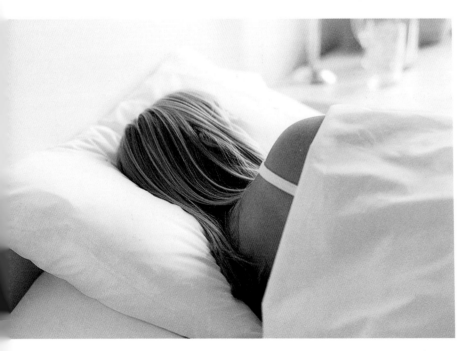

Never fall asleep without measuring your glucose level to check that it's stable and at the right level for you

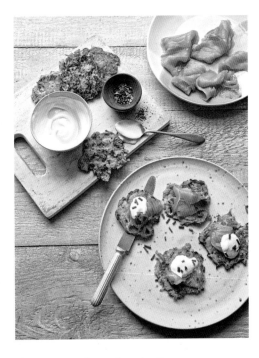

Eat balanced meals to keep your blood sugar happy, such as the Sweet Potato and Zucchini Pancakes on page 104.

in people under forty. "Dead in bed" is the term used when a person develops serious hypoglycemia while asleep and just never wakes up. You can imagine the fear that family and friends feel when their loved ones with diabetes go to sleep.

Ways to avoid being dead in bed include measuring your blood glucose before turning in for the evening and never falling asleep without having a level that is (1) stable (not trending downward) and (2) above a certain level (which is determined individually; for me it was above 110 mg/dL).

Another important piece of advice is to keep sugary snacks or power bars close to the bed—on the bedside table, for example. I also used to have a small snack before going to sleep, such as a few crackers or a piece of fruit together with a nice cup of tea. If you share your bed with someone, educate that person and provide him or her with tools to address a potential low, such as a glucagon pen and some sugar tablets.

Preventing dramatic lows

In recent years, an insulin pump that turns off when the sugar is below a certain level and does not turn on until two hours later has been approved and is on the market. This "hypo-shutoff" is the first step toward a closed-loop system, or as some people would call it, an artificial pancreas.

For all the people on insulin and using pumps, this is a major development, although we are far from safe yet, and much more research and capital need to go into this area of preventing people from going low. Another example of recent advances are the improved continuous glucose meters that make a sound when blood sugar is trending toward low levels, so you can eat something right away or get help from people who are with you. These glucose meters can also be connected wirelessly to cellular phones so that parents, spouses, or other loved ones can receive a text message when the person is going low.

Preventing dramatic lows is a primary goal for anyone living with diabetes. When your blood sugar is on its way down, your judgment and decision-making ability are compromised; you may not have timed your insulin perfectly with your exercise or had less to eat than normal. *Please* test your sugar and make sure it isn't trending downward.

Karin's story: *WHAT HAPPENS WHEN YOU GO LOW*

I remember vividly one of the times I went low, and it almost ended very badly. One day during the fall of 2007, I was walking on the beach in Westport, Connecticut, with my mother. The weather was still gorgeous. Because I was not wearing anything with pockets, I was not carrying any dextrose or food with me, thinking that I would be fine just taking a leisurely walk for thirty minutes.

I was testing a new insulin pump at the time— a pod pump, which delivered insulin continuously and was controlled by a remote device that increased, decreased, or completely turned off the insulin. I was still not used to it. Since my diagnosis, I had resisted wearing a pump and elected to use insulin pens instead, but I thought that this type of pump would give me more freedom than the pen, while still not being as bulky as traditional pumps.

On our way back to the car, I started to feel a little light-headed, and I quickly realized I was going low. I hesitated to tell my mother, but eventually I had to admit that I was not feeling well. She was worried and asked me if I had sugar in the car. I responded sheepishly that I had forgotten to bring anything. She went to get the car so that we could quickly drive back to the house to get me something sugary. I sat down on a bench to wait for her.

By that time I felt terrible. The whole world was spinning, I had broken out into a cold sweat, and my body shook uncontrollably. My vision was so blurred, I could hardly see, and I had a bad headache. I was consumed by fear, as I had been every time I had experienced a hypo. I felt as if I were in a tornado and being pulled into the eye of the storm. My mother returned with her car, and we drove back home faster than I have ever seen her drive (she is a very law-abiding citizen!). I remember arriving in the garage of my parents' house and my mother asking if I were still wearing the pump. I hardly heard her voice, which sounded as though it came from a different world, much less comprehended the significance of the question. She felt my upper arm and ripped off the pod pump. The next thing I recall is waking up on the kitchen sofa with a whole team of paramedics around me, an IV in my arm, and my parents hovering over me. I had been out for a significant amount of time, and only when the paramedics injected glucagon into my system as well as glucose through an IV did I regain consciousness.

I was taken to Norwalk Hospital, where I was treated for hypothermia, low blood pressure, and low heart rate by IV fluids, and I quickly felt much better. My adrenergic system (the system of organs and

This was an important reminder for me to carry
a snack with me at all times, even when I thought
it would not be needed

nerves that uses adrenaline and is responsible for the "fight or flight" reaction we have when faced with a threat) had kicked in; I was soaked in cold sweat and my body temperature was down to 93 degrees Fahrenheit (34 degrees Celsius). I could not stop shaking and crying. I had not just passed out, I had lost control of my body once again, and I required assistance to wake up. If I had been alone in my apartment in New York City, I would have died.

For some time afterward, I was scared every time I went to sleep. However, insulin pumps have become more sophisticated since then to avoid this kind of situation, and this episode was an important reminder for me to carry a snack with me at all times, even when I thought it would not be needed.

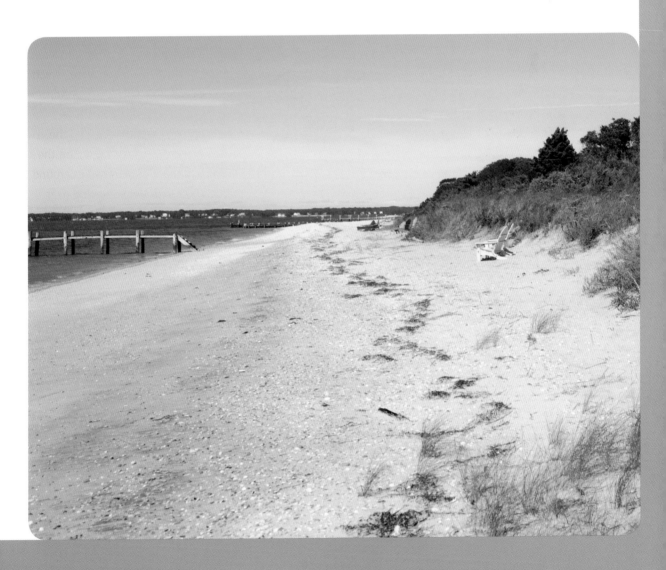

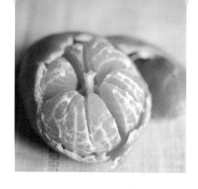

Keep sugary snacks or power bars on your bedside table, and have a small snack before going to sleep, such as a few crackers or a piece of fruit with a nice cup of tea

If you have diabetes, it is important to always keep sugary foods with you. Never leave your home without little bags of snacks, such as dextrose pills, a piece of fruit, or an energy bar. Pay attention to the signs of low blood sugar, and make sure your family and friends know what to look for as well. Telltale signs are headaches, shakiness, cold sweat, and blurred vision. Irritability and slurred speech are others. Going low can sometimes be mistaken for having consumed too much alcohol (another good reason to wear some sort of identification indicating that you have diabetes).

You want to avoid this state and prevent volatility in your blood sugar at all times. It is not good for you to have your blood sugar levels go up and down, so establishing a more stable glucose level, one you can safely live with, is important. Many studies have shown that having stable sugar levels is better than volatile levels when it comes to outcomes and complications.

REMEMBER

- For a person with diabetes, low blood sugar, or hypoglycemia, is a dangerous condition.

- Know the symptoms of low blood sugar and educate your family and friends about them as well.

- Always have dextrose tablets or sugary snacks with you, and try to avoid situations where you make yourself vulnerable to low blood sugar, such as going to bed without measuring your blood sugar and ensuring the levels are where they should be; exercising on an empty stomach; going for long hikes by yourself; and drinking alcohol without eating.

4 How to Eat

For people like me who live with diabetes, food is essential to our survival on several levels. What we feed our bodies supplies us with essential nutrients to sustain energy and hydration, and what we choose to eat can either nourish us or hurt us. But what and how we eat involves more than just basic physiology; there is a strong emotional aspect to eating with friends and family. Sharing a festive meal together can bring joy and support to all involved.

A culture of overeating and dieting

Children are not only urged to eat but are often encouraged by parents, relatives, or other people in authority to finish their meals (whether or not they're hungry), eat their vegetables, clean their plates, and not let anything go to waste. This is especially true for individuals growing up after hard times, such as wars, or when parents want to provide more for their children than they had when they were growing up.

This behavior makes sense during times of scarcity, which have occurred often in human history. Our bodies have learned to preserve energy and store it very efficiently. In fact, there are places in the world where people, like the Pima Indians of Arizona, have developed such a capacity for storing energy that they can survive for long periods of time with minimal nutrition.

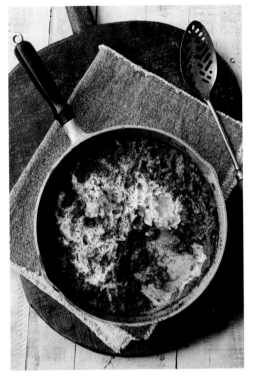

You can still eat delicious food as a diabetic—try the It's The Weekend Shakshuka on page 69.

However, in today's world, particularly in developed countries such as the United States, the recent availability of an ever-abundant food supply has triggered an incredibly high number of people suffering from obesity, insulin resistance, and diabetes. A constant wave of new, popular diets tells us that we need to lose a few pounds and that doing so will make us feel better and help us stay young. Every new theory creates a following of fans, and often the immediate results are impressive.

The reality is that although changing our behavior in the long term is hard, most people can implement a dramatic change for a short period of time. We have all heard about the Atkins Diet, the Juice Diet, the Lemon Diet, and the Caveman Diet, for example. There are numerous companies profiting from diet programs and food supplies. Currently, there is a lot of noise around smartphone applications that track food intake and recommend meals based on users' personal data and activity levels.

This all comes down to the basic energy equation: calories taken in cannot exceed what is being expended if we are not going to gain weight. Equally important is to maintain a *consistent* weight and to eat balanced meals with the right ratio of carbohydrates, fats, and proteins on some sort of regular schedule. The body is constantly burning calories to sustain its basic metabolic rate, even when we are sitting still or asleep. When we exercise or engage in other strenuous activities, our metabolism increases and we need more energy to maintain our strength. Children and adolescents, who are growing quickly, have a higher metabolic rate; they need more energy to build tissue, bones, and cells. For individuals with diabetes, the ability to break down nutrients or build up tissue may be affected by the disease or the drugs needed to combat the disease.

The effect of carbohydrates

Carbohydrates, such as fruit, bread, and pasta, are sources of energy. After digestive enzymes and the mechanics of the digestive tract break down a carbohydrate, the product is glucose. Glucose in the blood must be kept within a very narrow range, somewhere between 70 and 140 mg/dL; in a person who does not have diabetes, the blood sugar never exceeds 140 mg/dL, and the blood sugar never drops below 70 mg/dL, except in states of starvation. The hormones responsible for regulating the range of glucose in the blood are insulin and glucagon. We need glucose to enter the cells of our body to supply energy, but the only way it can be allowed into cells is through the action of insulin. Insulin is produced by the pancreas. When we eat a lot of carbohydrates, the pancreas needs to work very hard to produce more insulin.

When insulin levels are high, the glucose is converted not only into energy needed by the cells, but also into fat, which is stored in fatty tissue and around organs. This starts a vicious circle: the more fatty tissue in the body, the more insulin-resistant you become (i.e., the more insulin is needed to lower the same amount of glucose) and the harder the pancreas needs to work until it burns out, resulting in T2D.

Some doctors and dieticians recommend a very low-carb diet to lose weight, and the fact is that it works. When the body is forced to change its basic fuel from glucose to fats and proteins, weight loss occurs. However, not everyone can follow the diet because of food allergies, gastrointestinal issues, or just a general love for carbohydrates!

Because I have a transplanted pancreas, you may believe that I indulge in foods previously forbidden, but that is not the case. Maybe it is simply a habit, but I believe that the increased knowledge I have gained about high-sugar foods and drinks and refined carbohydrates continues to drive my lifestyle. I am a big fan of limiting simple carbs, such as sugar without fiber, white pasta, white rice, and potatoes. The last thing I want is to overtax and damage my new pancreas with unmanageable sugar loads.

Karin's story: *DANGER FOODS*

After I developed diabetes as a teenager, having a meal full of carbs was an ordeal. In fact, I avoided carbohydrates whenever I could during my years on insulin, especially after an incident in the summer of 1989. (Thanks to a successful pancreas transplant in 2010, I no longer need to take insulin.)

My diagnosis of T1D came only a few weeks before my parents, two sisters, and I moved to Paris. I welcomed the novelty of a new city, language, and routines. As a seventeen-year-old recently given a diagnosis of a chronic disease, I was happy to leave my old surroundings for a fresh start and new memories. In Paris, I could start going to a new school, build a life, and hide the disease from everyone but my doctors and immediate family. One evening, I had a normal, meal-sized portion of pizza—delicious, thin-crust pizza with tomato sauce, cheese, ham, and mushrooms. Later that evening, I woke up in agony. My skin felt too tight, I had a fever, and my head was bursting. I became agitated but at the same time started to feel drowsy, and my vision was blurred.

I had already established fairly tight routines of testing my blood sugar before and after meals and upon going to sleep and waking up, as well as dosing insulin to maintain a consistent blood glucose level. Although I had had a normal value before going to sleep, I decided to test my blood sugar, and lo and behold, the measurement was sky-high at 600 mg/dL! No wonder I felt so terrible. I was scared; I had already read about the negative consequences of poorly controlled diabetes, and I was determined to stay on top of my levels to avoid losing my

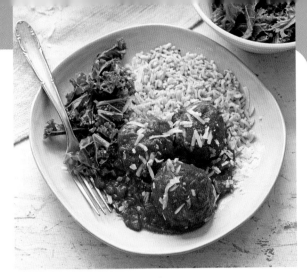

If you have carbohydrates with your meal, have them as a side and choose complex carbs—such as the Classic Meatballs with brown rice on page 90.

health to vision impairment, kidney failure, or nerve damage.

My elevated blood sugar was the result of a simple dinner of pizza. The white flour crust combined with a heavy helping of cheese and tomato sauce required much more insulin to digest than I had injected. I decided at that moment I would not expose myself to those kinds of reactions knowingly again, and I basically avoided pasta, pizza, white bread, pastries, rice, and potatoes for the next twenty-one years.

This was my choice, not that of my family or even my doctors. A common misconception is that diabetes patients can eat what they want as long as they dose their insulin correctly or even correct the dose after a meal if they indulge. In my view, it is easier to avoid these kinds of foods altogether, but that choice is obviously a personal one.

Eating at home

Today I indulge in low-carb meals that are high in lean protein and vegetable fats. I love fish and seafood, in particular grilled salmon, halibut, sea bass, and shrimp (prawns). I also love mushrooms of all kinds, especially sautéed or grilled. When I cook at home, these foods are always on the menu. I can eat an abundance of spinach and broccoli and feel satisfied yet not overfed.

Food makes me happy, gives me energy, and heats me up inside. I have never understood the joy of eating until you get drowsy and fall asleep. Perhaps my point of view comes from the time when those symptoms were correlated with high blood sugar, and I feared that feeling so very much I still relate it to danger rather than pleasure.

Snacking on nutrient-dense foods, such as nuts and fiber-rich fruits, is critical to keeping my energy level high enough to fuel my active life, which includes a demanding work schedule, international travel, daily exercise, and a satisfying social life.

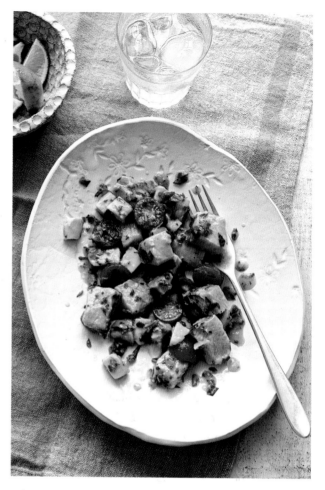

A favourite seafood dish of mine is the Salmon Ceviche on page 77.

Continue to celebrate holidays and festive occasions at the dining table. If you're eating at someone else's home, being open about your condition is essential, so that your host and hostess can plan a menu that will accommodate your diet as well as those of the other guests.

Take some time to read about healthful diets for people with diabetes. I have provided information on this in part 2 (see pages 50–59), along with a number of specially designed recipes. I think all people need to build their own approach together with their doctor and nutritionist, but as I have mentioned before, the key is to properly balance the energy equation (calories in should never exceed calories out) and to keep close control of carbohydrates. The healthful diet and lifestyle recommended for people with diabetes is actually optimal for everyone. We all benefit from fewer simple carbohydrates and more fiber, lean proteins, fats, and grains. This kind of diet can be delicious and nutritious. If we begin to think about the things we need to avoid and start to feel deprived, we are going down the wrong path and may end up making the wrong choices.

While carbohydrates are not forbidden, people with T2D should try to limit their consumption of them, since the pancreas has to work overtime to provide the insulin needed to keep the blood sugar within the normal range when carbs are eaten. If you have T1D, your insulin dose will need to be closely balanced with the carbs, and it is easier to keep your glucose levels stable if you moderate your consumption of carbohydrates.

Eating at restaurants

At a restaurant it is more difficult to control the eating experience. Still, I never have a problem asking a waiter to replace fried food with something broiled/grilled, steamed, or boiled or to substitute spinach, mushrooms, broccoli, or some lightly dressed greens for French fries and white rice. Many restaurants, even casual dining chains, make a point of having more healthful options on their menus. Don't feel bad about asking for these changes; you are the customer, and if they cannot accommodate your needs, you do not need to return, nor do you need to recommend this place to others. Your body is your engine, and just as you would not put inferior fuel into an expensive car, you should not put empty calories or unhealthful foods into your body. Remember that only you can manage your disease—no one else is ultimately responsible. Do not blame others for your dietary failures, your poor blood values, or your weight gain.

There are other, less obvious issues than food to consider when you're eating out. As an insulin-dependent person, you need to test your blood sugar before dosing insulin, whether you use a pump, pen, or syringe. It is difficult to plan your exact carb intake before you see the menu, so you will want to use the restaurant restroom to measure your blood sugar. (Not everyone is comfortable performing such a test at the table, followed by injecting insulin into their abdomen or thigh, nor may your dining companions or other guests be at ease with such procedures.) When I had to inject insulin, I always found the restaurant's ladies' room, since doing all this before leaving home would prove to be too early. Restaurants that lack proper restrooms are hard for people with diabetes. Optimally, the toilet and sink should be inside a booth so that there is privacy to perform these tasks.

Another important item is the timing of the food. When people with diabetes place their orders, they normally inject their insulin as well and have calculated the amount needed to cover their meal. If the first course takes too long to arrive, there may be a problem, since their blood sugar will start falling before the food has even been served. To avoid this, people with diabetes might give themselves their insulin before the food arrives or eat too much bread to eliminate the risk of going low. When I was on insulin, I would eat a little something before going out or ask the restaurant to quickly bring out some healthful snacks, such as crudités, cheese, or charcuterie. Clearly this is not possible in every restaurant, so having a small snack beforehand is wise.

Don't feel bad about asking for a more healthful option instead of the suggested side on the menu—you are the customer

Another important aspect of dining out is the restaurant's lighting and layout. Restaurants want to create an atmosphere, and I have been in a number of places where the lighting is low and there is a sudden step down or up. For a person who has had laser coagulation treatment to treat diabetic retinopathy, for example, it is difficult to quickly adjust to lighting changes, and unexpected steps can be a falling or tripping hazard. Even the path to the ladies' or men's rooms can be problematic. The restrooms are often on a higher or lower floor than the dining room, and the stairway and hall may not be well lighted. Last, the menu: in the best of all possible worlds it should be illuminated in some way or at least printed in large type to accommodate people with reduced vision, one of the complications of diabetes. Unfortunately, this is rarely the case. Carrying a miniature flashlight or a magnifier is quite helpful, but restaurants could also provide them, since in many cases people older than fifty who don't have diabetes need these kinds of tools as well!

! REMEMBER

- Eating is not just about fueling our bodies; it evokes strong emotions, brings families together, and is part of our culture. This can pose issues for people with diabetes since their state of mind may be very driven by blood sugar, which is related to food intake.

- It is important to maintain a healthy, consistent weight. The calories you consume cannot exceed the calories you expend.

- Eat a balance of lean protein, polyunsaturated fats, and a moderate amount of complex carbohydrates.

- Eat on a regular schedule: three meals and two snacks will keep your body fueled during the day.

- When eating at a restaurant or at someone else's home, don't be afraid to explain your condition so that your dietary restrictions can be accommodated.

5 Exercise and Diabetes

Exercising is important for the health of people with diabetes, and there is no doubt that exercise prolongs life and helps with the overall management of diabetes and other metabolic parameters. Exercise contributes to weight loss, and beyond the fact that we all want to look better, the less fatty tissue a person with diabetes has, the easier it is to manage sugar levels properly. The other benefits of exercise include reduced blood pressure, lower blood lipids, and an improved mood. Diet and exercise can actually reverse T2D in its early stages and prevent prediabetes from ever becoming diabetes.

How exercise affects blood sugar

Managing your blood sugar when exercising can be complicated. Exercise increases the uptake of glucose into the cells, reducing the need for insulin, which means your insulin dose needs to be reduced if you decide to play tennis or run after a meal. The metabolic

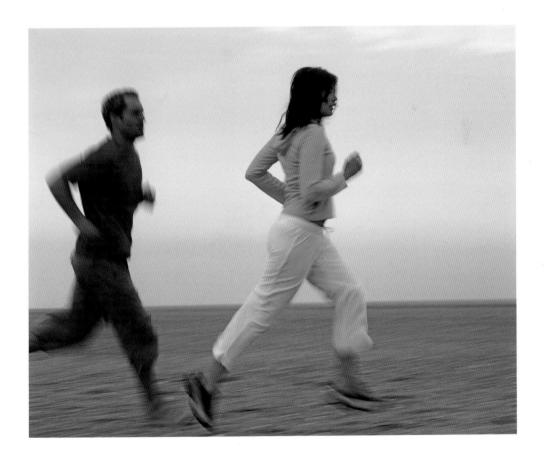

effects of exercise last after your activity is finished, so hours after exercise, glucose uptake can still be affected and your insulin dose must be adjusted.

When you exercise, the body uses two sources of fuel to generate energy: sugar and free fatty acids (fat). Sugar is stored in the liver and muscle in a form called glycogen. During the first fifteen minutes of exercise, most of the sugar for fuel comes from either the bloodstream or the muscle glycogen, which is converted back to sugar. After fifteen minutes of exercise, however, your body uses more of the glycogen stored in the liver. After thirty minutes of exercise, your body begins to get more of its energy from the free fatty acids. The body will replace the glycogen it has used, but this process may take four to six hours or even as long as twelve to twenty-four hours after more intense activity. While the body is rebuilding its glycogen stores, a person with diabetes can be at higher risk for hypoglycemia (see page 20).

Creating an exercise program after diagnosis

How you approach an exercise program will depend on whether you have T1D or T2D and how the disease is affecting you. Planning a program should be done with your doctor's okay and with help from a fitness professional who has experience working with people with diabetes. For a young person who has just received a diagnosis of T1D, the most important thing is to avoid hypos during and after working out, and to avoid exercise when in ketosis. For an adult with T2D who has metabolic syndrome (diabetes combined with overweight, high blood pressure, and blood lipid disturbances) and some late-stage complications, such as kidney or eye changes, any exercise program requires careful planning to determine what kind of exercise is allowed to avoid increasing his or her blood pressure too much or exerting the wrong effects on the heart and blood vessels.

I was an elite athlete when I received my diagnosis, and I knew nothing about

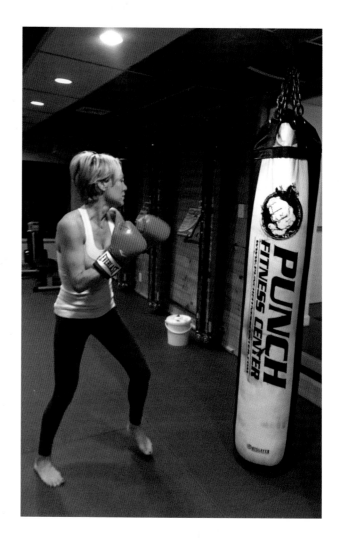

> Repetition and consistency are very important for results, and in the beginning it is critical to motivate yourself to exercise

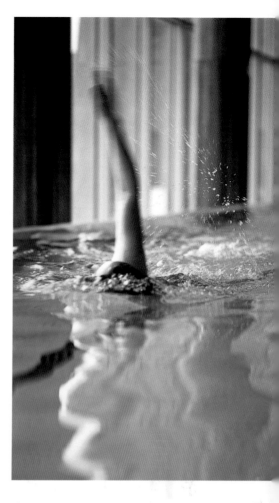

exercise other than pushing my body hard to the point of breakdown. I had to acknowledge that pursuing a professional tennis career would be much too hard. (There are a few examples of professional athletes with diabetes, such as Olympic gold medalist swimmer Gary Hall Jr, Olympic gold medalist rower Sir Steve Redgrave, and NFL star Jay Cutler, but there isn't an abundance of them.) There is a clear difference between performance sports and exercising simply to stay in shape, which is good for everyone. Even so, I love to be active, and my diabetes has definitely caused some trouble for me. To avoid nightly hypos, I do not exercise too late in the evening, and I have learned how to manage my sugars through well-planned snacks before and during my exercise sessions. Many times I have been frustrated when I had to stop a run or a tennis match because of going low.

Glucose management

Always measure your glucose level before any exercise, and follow these guidelines:

- lower than 100 mg/dL: The blood sugar may be too low to exercise safely. Eat a small carbohydrate-containing snack, such as fruit, before the workout.

- 100 to 250 mg/dL: For most people, this is a safe preexercise blood sugar range.

- 250 mg/dL or higher: Before exercising, test your urine for ketones. If you exercise when there is a high level of ketones you run the risk of ketoacidosis, a serious complication of diabetes that needs immediate treatment. Wait to exercise until there are no ketones detectable in the urine.

- 300 mg/dL or higher: The blood sugar is too high to exercise safely, as these high glucose levels may increase the risk of dehydration and ketoacidosis. Postpone the workout until the blood sugar drops to a safe preexercise range.

Diet and exercise can actually reverse Type 2 diabetes
in its early stages and prevent prediabetes from ever
becoming diabetes

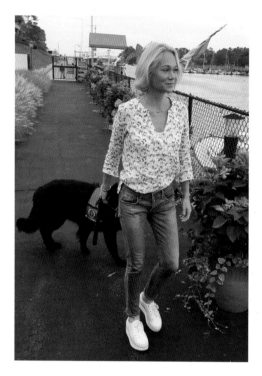

Building exercise into your life

Everyone with diabetes (and people without diabetes as well!) needs to move every day to speed up their metabolism, increase the glucose uptake into the cells, and build muscle. Muscle burns more energy than fat; the more muscle you have, the more efficient and effective your metabolism becomes.

Making exercise part of your everyday routine is key. Repetition and consistency are very important for results, and in the beginning it is critical to motivate yourself. One method I have found that works well is recording your food intake and exercise program, either manually or through electronic bio tools. I have tried the Fitbit, the Nike+ FuelBand, and the Jawbone, and they all serve a purpose. They won't make you exercise and they won't give you a present if you go to the gym, but it is quite nice to see the number of steps you have taken each day and compare your accomplishments to your history or someone else's. The other strong motivator is the weighing scale, in addition to other body measurements that are affected by your fitness. I used to hate the scale, but if you weigh yourself daily, you can quickly catch a dangerous trend, either upward or downward.

Joining a gym can help you create a helpful exercise regime. However, many gyms are intimidating to people with a disability or who are not very physically fit. Choosing the right gym is especially important for people with a chronic disease such as diabetes. Similar to restaurants, the layout and the facilities should be adjusted to accommodate those who may have difficulties with their vision. Most important, all trainers and personnel should have a basic understanding of diabetes and what to do if someone goes low. There are some specialized gyms catering solely to people with diabetes. One of those is called Fitscript and is based in Connecticut. I encourage you to look them up and learn from the lessons they are providing about exercise and diabetes.

A typical day for me involves an hour-long, brisk walk-run in the morning with my dog. I love these walks: they wake me up, get me moving in the fresh air, and set the pace for the day. I normally listen to music while I run or walk, and I try to sprint intervals between jogging and walking. During the day, either at work or at home, there are always opportunities to break away for a little workout, like walking around the block, jogging up the stairs, or, if there is a gym on the premises, getting some aerobic and weight exercise. At the end of the day and after any meal, walking and using your muscles (you could do some sit-ups or push-ups or even work out with some light weights) will help greatly with digestion and blood sugar control. The worst thing you can do is to lie down for a siesta after a meal.

I still love a good hour of tennis, kickboxing, or a core class, but as long as I continue the basic program I described above, I maintain my metabolic health and overall well-being. I strongly encourage you to exercise. Your own program does not have to include complicated classes or expensive training programs. It can merely be walking forty-five to sixty minutes daily and doing a few sets of sit-ups at home. There are benefits to cross-training and increasing your heart rate regularly, but for a person with little experience who is not particularly fit, simple walks and sit-ups can do the trick.

! REMEMBER

• Exercise helps with the overall management of diabetes, contributing to weight loss. Other benefits include reduced blood pressure, lower blood lipids, and improved mood.

• Diet and exercise can actually reverse T2D in its early stages and prevent prediabetes from ever becoming diabetes.

• Planning an exercise program should be done with your doctor's okay and with help from a fitness professional who has experience working with people with diabetes.

• Test your blood sugar levels before beginning to exercise.

• Move every day to speed up your metabolism, increase the glucose uptake into your cells, and build muscle.

6 Traveling and Vacations

Going away for the holidays or taking a vacation is therapeutic for the body and the mind. The mind needs a break from daily routines, and much research has shown that efficiency in the workplace can be improved when people are rested and happy. However, a person with diabetes can never take a vacation from the disease.

In the mountains, by the water—wherever you choose to go for a change of pace and atmosphere—you still have to monitor and treat your diabetes. This can be a hard fact to accept, and many people find it unfair that they are not allowed to break the rules sometimes. The reality is that short-term deviations from your routine diet and exercise plan probably do not cause much long-term damage, but the immediate consequences are most often not worth the pleasure. Neither going high, which means having a blood sugar level that is higher than normal, nor going low is exactly a pleasant feeling, but it is not wrong to indulge in a gourmet meal once in a while as long as you make sure to adjust your insulin dose or exercise levels accordingly.

What to consider

Certain venues and activities are better than others for people with a chronic disease. For example, an isolated location or a developing country may not have the necessary medical facilities to accommodate you, should an emergency arise. And obviously you should know the location of the nearest medical facility and have access to nutritious food and clean water.

For diseases such as diabetes, the dosing of the medication must be timely and that can be a problem when one travels across time zones. The fast-acting insulin is dosed according to when you eat, but there is also the long-acting insulin that normally is dosed before bedtime, and in some cases is needed twice daily. I noticed, especially when traveling across the Atlantic, that I had to carefully adjust my doses, since the circadian rhythm is disrupted and the time I was active versus resting was essentially reversed. This is much easier done with a pump, using continuously delivered insulin. The basal rate can almost always just continue as is, while one simply adjusts the bolus doses to when the meals are being served. However, it is quite common that the blood sugar levels run a little less steady during the trip and for a few days in the new time zone.

Before you go on any kind of trip, do some research about the hotel, city, and neighborhood before committing to any plans. You want to make sure there is good care available if something happens. It is not worth risking your life for an exotic location, in my opinion. My second piece of advice is to teach travel companions what your symptoms are when you are low or high. If they can spot the shakiness, irritability, and cold sweat before you

In the mountains, by the water—wherever you choose to go for a change of pace and atmosphere—you still have to monitor and treat your diabetes

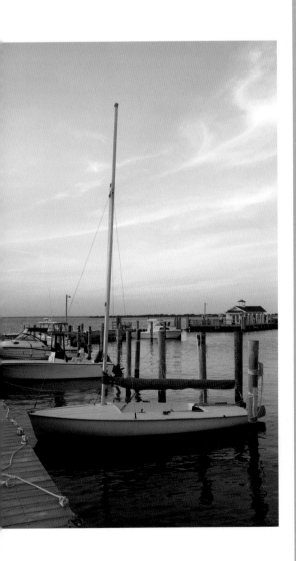

Karin's story: *LEARNING FROM EXPERIENCE*

I made a few mistakes when traveling while having T1D, one of which was not telling people around me that I had the disease. This meant that no one accommodated my need for regular meals and snacks. I was forced to reduce my insulin injections to avoid going low, and I ended up being too high most of the time as a consequence. Forgetting your equipment is another risk not advised. I remember one wedding I went to with my then fiancé; I got a stomach bug and had to be treated with IV fluids. I had forgotten my glucose meter, and I was very scared that I did not know my sugar values while I was unable to keep down any food or fluids. This was obviously a perilous situation, since blood sugar can become dangerously low very quickly. When you travel, you must be clear about your condition and the management it requires. Also, make sure you have your equipment! Both these things should be on the to-do list of every person with diabetes. Another experience was when I flew to the US from Sweden and had not brought my own food on the plane. I dosed my insulin, but then when the food service arrived, I realized there was nothing on the tray I wanted to eat, so I ended up going low during the flight. This is not a pleasant episode, since flying by itself can be stressful, and having to deal with hypoglycemia as well is not something you want to add. I ended up being okay, but from then on, I always brought fruit, some crackers, and an energy bar onboard a plane to avoid going low.

Short-term deviations from your routine diet and exercise plan probably do not cause much long-term damage, but the immediate consequences are most often not worth the pleasure

do, they can make sure you get something to eat and prevent a catastrophic event. Carry snacks with you, and ask your companions to do so also. Consider packing an extra set of equipment to be on the safe side. Insulin is a protein and needs to be kept cool. When it is in the pen, syringe, or pump, you can store it at room temperature, but only for a limited amount of time. The extra supplies in vials that must be brought for longer trips need to be stored in a refrigerator. Proteins denature in the sun, which could explain random high glucose levels, since it would render the insulin less potent. It is very important to have a doctor's note saying that you have diabetes and must travel with insulin and testing supplies, especially if you are flying. Transportation Security Administration regulations do not apply to medical supplies, but you don't want to risk having yours confiscated.

Otherwise, my recommendations are pretty similar to those for anyone traveling: be careful, enjoy, relax, and come back refreshed!

REMEMBER

- You can take (and enjoy!) a vacation, but you cannot take a vacation from diabetes.

- Make sure you are aware of the nearest medical facility at your destination.

- Pack snacks and make sure you and your companions carry them at all times.

- Carrying extra equipment and insulin is always a good idea. Travel with a doctor's note saying that you have diabetes and need injectable insulin. This is especially important if you are traveling by airplane.

7　Your Relationships

So far I have mentioned only the physical aspects of living with diabetes, but there is also a big psychological component to deal with, both for people with diabetes and for their partners and other loved ones. Having a chronic disease automatically means the person with the condition requires more attention than an average individual, and that can be difficult both for those with diabetes and for their partners. Living with the fear of complications is another aspect of the psychology of diabetes, and a good partner must deal with that in a positive and constructive way.

Having a partner you can trust through thick and thin is the ultimate goal for most of us, and it is truly a privilege when it happens. People with a chronic illness such as diabetes may end up getting hurt by, and breaking up with, people who just are not ready for the commitment it takes. Many young couples do not need to test the "hard times" until later in life; it takes a special person to live with someone who may require help managing their condition. People with diabetes, however healthy they are, do need to seek more medical attention than the average person, and they need to pay more careful attention to their food and exercise.

Trying to establish the right relationship of trust and love when you are a young adult can be hard enough when you are still developing as a person and trying to fit in. Having a chronic disease adds another layer of complexity to the equation. The younger and more inexperienced we are, the more selfish we are (in my opinion), and a potential partner may not want to take on the responsibility of a "sick" person.

Learning to trust

Romantic relationships were secondary to my education, and later, to my job. My sisters, my parents, and my close friends have always been my safety net. I moved a lot for work, and although on the plus side, constant relocation taught me how to adjust quickly in new groups and develop friendships in different communities, it also taught me never to rely on anyone being there for the long haul, except for my immediate family.

Having a chronic, potentially debilitating disease presented many hurdles when it came to forming friendships and romantic attachments, some that were real and some that my imagination built up to be larger than they should have been. Since I was not open about having diabetes, I could not be completely honest with my friends. When it came to romantic relationships, I was careful too. I thought a potential partner would discard me immediately if he knew I had a disease that could make me unconscious at times, a disease that limited my food choices and required me to inject insulin into my abdomen.

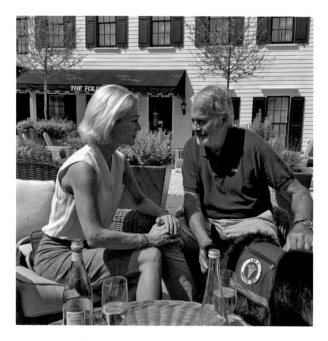

If you have diabetes, it is much better to be honest about your physical and emotional challenges—do not hesitate to ask for help

My mood was also affected by the sugar swings. But since people did not know, they could not easily understand why I would get irritable when I needed to eat, and they often thought I was picky when it came to my food choices.

I used to avoid telling new friends about my disease until I thought they were going to be around for a while and that they were people with whom I wanted to build a sustained friendship or romantic connection. That way I didn't have to see their reaction to my diabetes before I had a chance to win them over. In most cases, I elected to leave people in the dark, never letting them in on my deepest secret, what I considered a defect. It is almost impossible to get really close to someone without sharing details of how you feel physically on a daily basis or what your long-term fears are. When I did speak about what I had to go through, I was surprised to find that people's reactions were not negative. Misunderstandings actually occurred when I did not explain why I followed a stricter-than-normal diet or why I had to excuse myself before meals to test my blood sugar and inject insulin.

There were times after I received my new kidney and pancreas when men disappointed me. Instead of being happy that I was healthy again, one man I dated told me that he did not dare to fall in love with me since he would get hurt if I became extremely ill or died prematurely. I am sure this was just a line he used to tell me that he was not interested in anything serious, but regardless, it hurt. Needless to say, the relationship did not last. Another man told me that he did not have the energy to get involved with someone who may require extra help, and I quickly let him go since I would have been reluctant and afraid of showing weakness.

However, a relationship can grow into something better and more fulfilling through honesty. One man told me that I should consider myself very fortunate to be the recipient of one of my father's kidneys and the pancreas of a young woman who had passed away. He made me realize that I am one of the fortunate ones and that feeling sorry for myself is futile. I wake up each morning thinking about that and thanking the people who made it possible from the bottom of my heart. Over time, this man proved himself to be very strong and supportive, even when I was at my worst. Going through scary situations that are foreign to someone who is not used to sick people can either break or build a relationship. This man helped me in a way that was not patronizing, nor was he dismissive. He managed to hit the right balance and find the exact words and actions to make me feel cared for but not weak. It made the relationship grow and gave me more confidence in him.

Be honest

If you have diabetes, it is much better to be honest about your physical and emotional challenges. Do not hesitate to ask for help. You also need to realize that your partner will have his or her own fears and struggles about your condition and that you need to be sensitive to him or her too.

If you are the friend or loved one of someone with diabetes, it can be hard to strike a balance between letting that person be independent and being overprotective because you understand and are concerned about the challenges of his or her condition. Honesty and clear communication are important in all relationships; for a person with diabetes, they are essential.

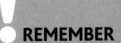

REMEMBER

• Having a chronic illness such as diabetes can affect your friendships and romantic relationships.

• Diabetes presents psychological and emotional challenges as well as physical ones.

• It is important to be open and honest with your friends and loved ones about your condition and your special needs.

8 Living on Your Own

Leaving your parents' house for college or moving into your first apartment is an exciting—and maybe a little scary—rite of passage. For someone with diabetes, it is an even bigger step toward independence, because you are now responsible not only for your own laundry and food, but also for managing your diabetes. When you were living at home, your parents may have been the ones supervising your medical care, including making doctors' appointments, picking up drugs, overseeing your medication, and monitoring your food and exercise. Now this is all your responsibility.

Weight gain and alcohol

Young adults often gain (most common) or lose a lot of weight during their first year at college. It's up to you when and what you eat; late-night snacks while studying and eating on the run can pack on the pounds. For the kid without diabetes, this just means buying some new clothes, but if you have diabetes, gaining weight can wreak havoc on your health. As I have said before, weight management is an important factor in managing diabetes, and the eating habits you establish when you're living alone for the first time can affect your health in the long term, for good or for ill.

For people with diabetes, no matter what their age, drinking too much is very dangerous. It is particularly problematic for someone who is inexperienced and does not know his or her limits. When you drink, your liver can break down the alcohol or balance low blood sugar by converting glycogen into glucose; it cannot do both at the same time. When the

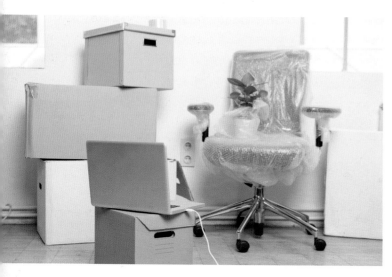

For someone with diabetes, leaving your parents' house means you are now responsible not only for your own laundry and food, but also for managing your diabetes

Karin's story: ASKING FOR HELP

When I moved away from home to attend medical school, I lived by myself for the first time. I was not an experienced cook and mostly ate yogurt or soup for dinner, though I did get nutritious lunches at school. I lost a tremendous amount of weight that first year (stress made me less likely to snack or eat heavy meals), but in my second year, I stabilized and kept a healthy weight. I did find a very competent physician who kept track of my metabolic state. I remember a number of instances at school when I started feeling low and quickly found a secluded spot where I could test my sugar and eat a snack. I was very uncomfortable sharing my story; instead, I took on the full burden of managing my diabetes myself. I do not recommend this! My fellow students and professors could have offered help and support rather than wondering why I sometimes disappeared or was picky about my food.

I moved to Boston after I completed medical school, my PhD, and my clinical internship. I was going for a post-doc at Harvard in what could be described as a very stressful environment. My family lived a few hours away, but I was living by myself and not interested in getting help. I was tired of managing the diabetes and became very careless for a period of time. This choice was damaging to my system, and my blood sugar values quickly got out of control. My weight plummeted, not because of excessive dieting or exercise, but because my blood sugar levels were constantly running too high. This was no one's fault but my own.

The reality is that most people want to forget about their disease once in a while. Since diabetes

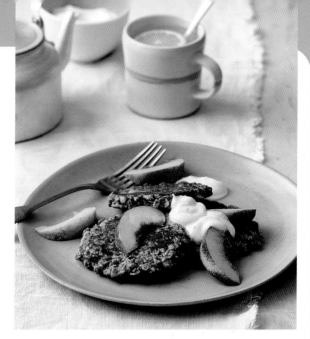

Eating well can be challenging when first living on your own, but learning simple recipes, such as the Pr-OAT-ein Pancakes on page 65, will stand you in good stead.

has terrible short-term consequences when the blood sugar is low and awful but long-term consequences when the blood sugar is maintained too high, it is easier to run high and not think about the future. However, if this strategy is implemented for a long period of time, you will most likely pay dearly for your lack of control. With a young person, this is often the case, not only in regards to diabetes, but smoking, drinking, etc., all fall under the same behavior pattern. When you are twenty-five years of age, it is hard to think about struggling with eye disease and kidney failure ten years later.

liver is busy metabolizing alcohol, your glucose can easily drop to dangerously low levels. If this situation is combined with a loss of awareness or even consciousness, you may not recognize that you're experiencing hypoglycemia.

Do your research

If you are living on your own for the first time, investigate your new environment carefully beforehand. Identify a doctor with expertise in your condition and make an appointment, or go to the school clinic and make sure they have your medical history. Know where to buy healthy food and where to exercise. It is important to confide in a few people—your roommate(s), close friends, perhaps your teachers—so that they know how to react if you start feeling bad. Try to establish routines early on, and do not forget your old ones. You do not have to completely change your habits just because you are moving away from your family. Some of the things you did at home can easily be transferred to the new environment with a little adjustment.

!

REMEMBER

• Going away to college or moving into your own apartment may be the first time you are solely responsible for managing all aspects of your diabetes.

• Staying at a healthy weight by eating well and exercising is very important to maintaining stable blood sugar values.

• Drinking heavily could make your blood sugars drop to dangerously low levels.

• Focus on the long term, and try to avoid falling into the trap of living dangerously just because you are young and invincible.

• When you arrive at your college or new apartment, find a doctor. Take note of where you can get nutritious food and exercise.

• Tell key people—your roommate(s), close friends, and perhaps your teachers—about your diabetes.

9 Looking Good

Everyone loves the idea of having a toned body, flawless skin, and shiny, healthy hair. Whether we are blond like Freya, the mythical Nordic goddess, or have black hair like Cleopatra, the Egyptian queen, we all look better when we are healthy, and we feel stronger when we look good! Looks—although we may want to believe they are secondary—can affect our confidence and even our attitude toward life. I believe strongly that a healthy body is beautiful and that people respond positively to you when you look and feel good.

Staying hydrated

Diabetes can affect the way you look as well as the way you feel. We have all heard how important it is to hydrate properly, both by consuming enough water daily and using moisturizers on our skin. Unstable blood sugar can result in chronic dehydration, which is bad for the skin and hair. If your blood glucose is high, your body loses fluid, and you urinate more to remove excess glucose from the blood, which causes your skin to become dry. Your skin can also get dry if the nerves, especially those in your legs and feet, do not get the message to sweat because of diabetic neuropathy (nerve damage). Sweating helps keep your skin soft and moist. Don't forget the basics: drink copious amounts of water and slather your skin with moisturizer. Also, avoid getting sunburned (which is a good idea for everyone!).

Unstable blood sugar can result in chronic dehydration, which is bad for the skin and hair: drink copious amounts of water and slather your skin with moisturizer

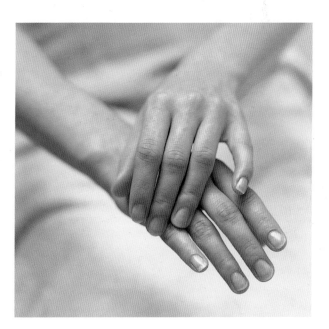

Other skin problems

Some specific conditions can occur in diabetes that require medical intervention, such as poor blood supply to peripheral tissues—the skin on your feet and ankles, for example—that could lead to poor healing of wounds and loss of sensitivity to injury. Dry skin can become red and sore or crack and peel. Dry skin can also be itchy, and scratching can lead to breaks in the skin. Germs can enter through the cracks in your skin and cause an infection. Excess glucose provides an excellent breeding ground for bacteria and fungi and can reduce the body's ability to heal itself.

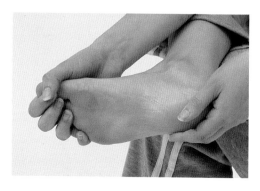

All these factors put people with diabetes at greater risk for skin problems, both mild and more serious. In fact, the American Diabetes Association says that as many as a third of people with diabetes will have a skin disorder related to their disease at some time in their lives. Fortunately, most skin conditions can be prevented and successfully treated if caught early. But if not cared for properly, a minor skin condition can turn into a more serious problem with potentially severe consequences. You would be wise to seek out a great dermatologist. Taking care of your skin is important for your overall well-being; it is the largest organ of the body and, if damaged, can cause serious physical and psychological consequences.

Looking after your feet

Keep your feet happy! It's a good idea to see a podiatrist. Get regular pedicures, but make sure you go to a salon with impeccable standards of cleanliness. If your nerves are damaged, you may not feel pain fully if you are nicked or cut and a pedicure could cause more damage than good. Wear comfortable, supportive shoes when walking long distances. Pay attention to your socks too. You do not want socks that rub against the skin and cause damage, so use soft ones with less elastic to prevent them from restricting the blood supply. I am very careful when I get manicures and pedicures. I do not allow knives near my feet, and I make sure that the place is clean and well organized. The same goes for any beauty treatment, including hair and makeup services.

Concealing diabetic equipment

Diabetes comes with a lot of "stuff" to be carried around. Some of it, such as pumps and continuous blood glucose monitors, is even attached to your body. This can make it harder to wear clothes that are fitted or more revealing. For example, girls and women may feel awkward displaying their pumps while they are wearing a form-fitting dress or while on the beach in a bathing suit. Concealing equipment may be a little easier for men, since they often have pockets, and their clothes cover more of their bodies and are usually looser. People have experimented with various solutions, such as a halter for the pump or meter around the thigh under an evening dress, and it is possible to disconnect your equipment for short periods of time if you are going for a swim. The patch pump is an improvement, since it is untethered and thus has no tubing to get caught. But even that needs to sit somewhere and cannot easily be hidden during the summer. There are companies out there trying to cover up these devices, as can be done for IV insertion lines, but nothing works perfectly yet.

Looking good will make you smile. It is fun to shop for new clothes, especially if your body is in good shape; that could be your reward for following a healthy diet and exercise program. The more than 110 million people in both the United States and the UK living with diabetes and prediabetes need more than just medical care. The whole person needs to be considered, and that includes skin, hair, fashion, and flair! I have seen how companies are trying to make it easier for people with chronic diseases, and I recently saw a great website for women who have completed breast cancer treatments. They focus on the nonmedical items patients search for and try to make the site a complete "marketplace" to simplify shopping for women and their relatives during a time when they may not have the energy to search all over the Internet for solutions.

REMEMBER

● You look better when you feel better. Good looks can give you confidence and improve your attitude toward life. Healthy is beautiful!

● Hydrate and moisturize! The skin of people with diabetes requires special care: dry, cracked skin can lead to infections.

● It is important to take care of your feet.

● Sometimes pumps and glucose meters make dressing a challenge, but there are creative solutions.

● Creating curated one-stop shopping sites for specific conditions would simplify the shopping experience of those living with a chronic disease.

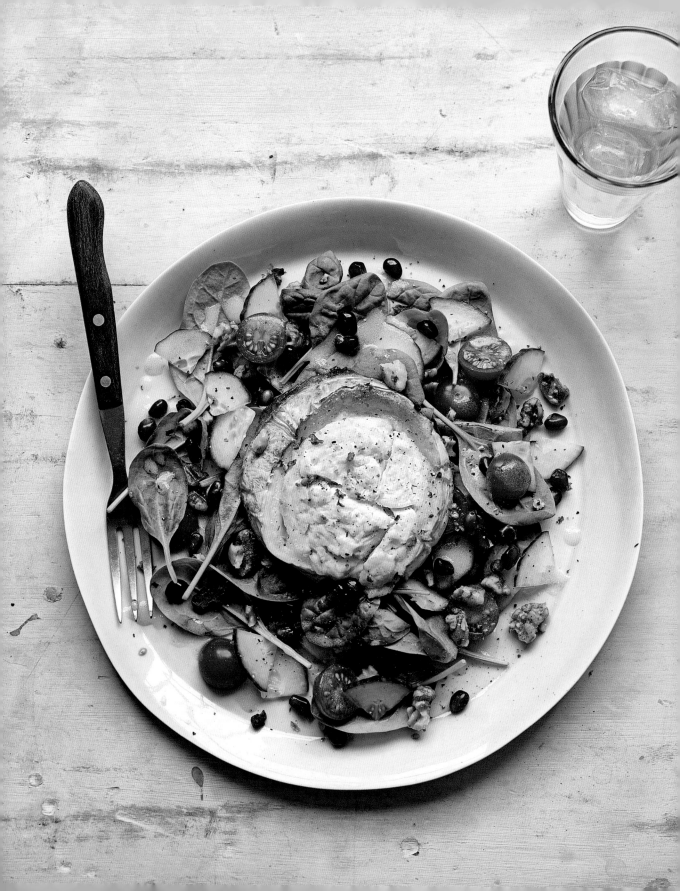

PART 2: The Recipes

Nutrition and Weight Loss

It has clearly been established that nutrition plays a major role in the treatment and management of diabetes. In T2D it may even be a way to reverse the disease at its earliest stages, by reducing insulin resistance peripherally and thus alleviating the pancreas from having to produce extra insulin and eventually tiring out completely, which would render the person insulin dependent.

Nutrition has a major role in the management of T1D, but it cannot reverse the condition, due to the fact that T1D is an autoimmune disease (see page 10). A person with diabetes should thus be very aware of what they eat and make sure they receive all their nutritional needs while not overindulging in foods that can affect their metabolic parameters—these are the measurable factors that define metabolism, such as glucose or lipids (which are blood fats, including cholesterol)—negatively and over-exert the pancreas.

A healthy diet for people with T1D and T2D

Nutritional recommendations for people with diabetes need to be personalized, and this is something you would discuss with your medical team (see page 18). However, the overall goals are to:

1 Attain and maintain the following:

- Blood glucose levels in the normal range, or as close to normal as is safely possible, to prevent or reduce the risk for complications of diabetes.

- Levels of blood fats, including cholesterol, that reduce the risk for disease of the large blood vessels (macrovascular disease).

- Blood pressure levels that reduce the risk for blood vessel disease.

2 Modify nutrient intake and lifestyle as appropriate for the prevention and treatment of the chronic complications of diabetes, including obesity, imbalance of blood fats (such as high cholesterol), heart disease, high blood pressure, and kidney disease.

3 Improve health through healthy food choices and physical activity.

4 Address individual nutritional needs, taking into consideration personal and cultural preferences and lifestyle while respecting the individual's wishes and willingness to change.

Proteins, fats, and carbohydrates

Basic nutrition includes an understanding of what the different food groups are, but before even discussing the food groups, we must understand what proteins, fats, and carbohydrates do for energy generation in the human body.

Proteins, fats, and carbohydrates provide 90 percent of the dry weight of the diet and 100 percent of its energy. They supply different amounts of energy (measured in calories, also known as kcal):

1 oz protein provides 112 calories / 25 g protein provides 100 calories
1 oz fat provides 252 calories / 25 g fat provides 225 calories
1 oz carbohydrate provides 112 calories / 25 g carbohydrate provides 100 calories

They also dispense energy at different rates; carbohydrates are the quickest, and fats are the slowest.

Proteins, fats, and carbohydrates are digested in the intestine, where they are broken down into their basic units:

Proteins are broken down into amino acids.
Fats are broken down into fatty acids and glycerol.
Carbohydrates are broken down into sugars.

Proteins

Proteins are used to build new proteins with specific functions, such as catalyzing chemical reactions, facilitating communication between different cells, or transporting biological molecules from one place to another. When there is a shortage of fats or carbohydrates, proteins can also yield energy.

Food that are high in protein include meat, fish, chicken, and some vegetables such as beans and nuts.

Fats

Fats typically provide more than half of the body's energy needs. Fatty acids that aren't needed right away are packaged in bundles called triglycerides and stored in fat cells, which have unlimited capacity. The human body is really good at storing fat.

Food that are high in fat include butter, cream, lard, avocados, nuts, certain seafood, and olive oil.

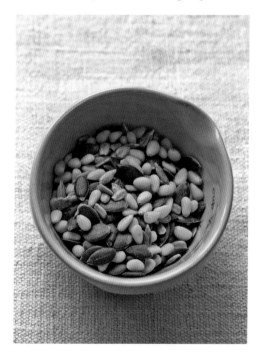

Nuts and seeds, such as pumpkin and sunflower seeds, are high in protein.

Carbohydrates

Carbs are much more difficult to store; in fact, we can only store a day or two's worth of carbs, and once the cells have been satisfied with glucose, the liver stores some of the excess for distribution between meals should blood glucose levels fall below a certain threshold. If there is leftover glucose beyond what the liver can hold, it can be turned into fat for long-term storage so none is wasted. When carbohydrates are scarce, the body runs mainly on fats. If energy needs exceed those provided by fats in the diet, the body must liquidate some of its fat tissue for energy.

Some types of cells, such as brain cells, have special needs. These cells can easily run on glucose from the diet, but they can't run on fatty acids directly. So under low-carbohydrate conditions, these cells need the body to make fat-like molecules called ketone bodies. This is why a very-low-carbohydrate diet is sometimes called "ketogenic." (Ketone bodies are also related to a dangerous diabetic complication called ketoacidosis, which can occur if insulin levels are far too low—see page 14.) Ketone bodies could alone provide enough energy for the parts of the body that can't metabolize fatty acids, but some tissues still require at least some glucose, which isn't normally made from fat. Instead, glucose can be made in the liver and kidneys using protein from elsewhere in the body, but the body will start chewing on muscle cells if not enough protein is provided by the diet.

Foods that are high in carbs include bread, rice, potatoes, pasta, fruit, and, of course, candy, cookies, and cakes.

Food groups and the diabetes food pyramid

There are five food groups: vegetables and legumes; fruits; grains; lean meats, including poultry, fish, eggs, tofu, nuts, and seeds; and, finally, milk and other dairy products (excluding cheese). A food pyramid is a way of representing the ideal number of servings for each food group that an individual should eat each day, with more servings of the food at the bottom of the pyramid and fewer at the top. For a person with diabetes, the food pyramid needs to be organized a little differently because it groups foods based on their carbohydrate and protein content instead of their classification as a food.

The diabetes food pyramid, shown opposite, takes into account the carb content in some of the dairy products, legumes, and grains. For example, milk and cheese are separated, where milk is organized into carb-containing foods, while cheese belongs with meats. Starchy and non-starchy veggies are distributed similarly, with the starchy ones included in the carb section. Portion size is also determined by carb content, allowing 1/2 oz (15 g) of carbs in any one carb choice.

The exact number of servings you need depends on your diabetes goals, calorie and nutrition needs, your lifestyle, and the foods you like to eat. Divide the number of servings you should eat among the meals and snacks you eat each day.

The diabetes food pyramid
This diagram shows the food groups and the ideal daily servings of each type for a person with diabetes.

FATS, OILS, AND SWEETS

Use sparingly

This group includes potato chips (crisps), fried foods, candy, cookies, and cakes. Make servings small and have them as an occasional treat.

MILK AND YOGURT

2–3 servings per day

Choose non-fat and low-fat options to avoid saturated fats. Those who are lactose intolerant could choose fortified soy milk, rice milk, or almond milk.

LEAN MEAT, MEAT SUBSTITUTE, AND OTHER PROTEINS

4–6 oz (110–170 g) per day, divided between meals

As well as meat and fish, this group includes eggs, tofu, cheese, cottage cheese, peanut butter, nuts, and seeds.

VEGETABLES AND LEGUMES

3–5 servings per day

Non-starchy vegetables are those not included in the grains and other starches group, such as carrots, broccoli, spinach, lettuce, and cucumber.

FRUITS

2–4 servings per day

The best choices of fruit are fresh, frozen, or canned (avoid those with added sugar). You may also choose dried fruit or fruit juice (not from concentrate), but the portion sizes are small, so they may not be as filling.

GRAINS AND OTHER STARCHES

6–11 servings per day

This includes bread, rice, pasta (but avoid white varieties of these) and cereal—foods that are made mostly of grains, such as wheat, rye and oats. It also includes starchy vegetables, such as potatoes, peas, corn, and dry beans (for example, pinto beans and lentils).

Making the right choices

Breakfast

- Coffee or tea (with no addition of milk or sugar) speed up your metabolism and may lower the blood sugar and decrease your weight. There is no need to add insulin.

- Yogurt or milk with cereal is high in carbs, especially if you choose a cereal that includes sugar.

- Oatmeal is also high in carbs, but it contains fiber, which delays the sugar peak somewhat and actually helps you sustain energy for a period of time.

- Toast with butter is VERY high in fast-acting carbs, which makes it unsuitable for someone with brittle diabetes (a special kind of diabetes that is hard to regulate). The combination of carbs and the surface of the toasted bread for some reason make the sugar spike even more than if eating regular bread that is not toasted.

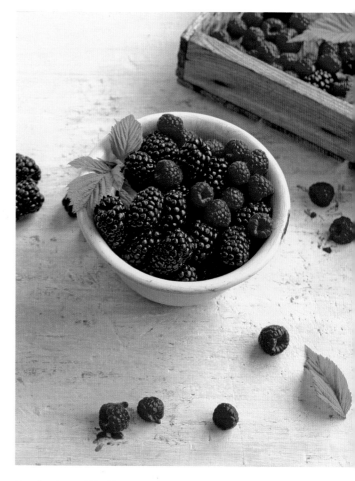

Raspberries and blackberries are high in fiber and vitamin C.

- Eggs, avocados, cheese, ham, and turkey are all good breakfast items for people with diabetes since they contain protein and fat but have a very low carb content.

- Fruits are high in simple carbohydrates, but are a better option than processed sugars. Some fruits are better than others, for example, berries are recommended for people with diabetes.

Lunch

- Salads made with leafy greens, green veggies, and some lean protein, such as tuna, chicken, or turkey, are a great alternatives to sandwiches, the lunch option most often served in corporate settings.

- I avoid a lunch based on bread, but it is okay occasionally to eat a sandwich made with whole wheat bread and filled with some lean protein.

- Equally, one slice of multigrain toast or even a side order of brown rice with your lunch will provide complex carbs for sustained energy.

Dinner

- Broiled/grilled or sautéed fish with veggies is a great low-carb dish for people with diabetes or anyone who wants to lose weight.

- Use a spiralizer or vegetable peeler to create noodles or ribbons from zucchini (courgettes) or other non-starchy vegetables to use in place of wheat pasta.

- Try to eat dinner earlier rather than later; eight o'clock should be your cut-off time. In fact, late dinners are bad for everyone.

- It is never good to eat a heavy carb meal at the end of the day if you want to lose weight. Have fewer carbs for dinner than you did for breakfast and lunch, since you are on your way to ending the day and do not want carbs to disturb your sleep (because of volatile blood sugar) or make you gain weight if you don't exercise after dinner.

- At the same time, however, it is also actually quite important for a diabetic to eat some carbs before going to bed, since you want to avoid "going low" in your sleep. I would test my blood sugar prior to going to sleep, and if it was not above a certain number, I would eat a piece of fruit, a few crackers, or even a cookie! This is not recommended for people with diabetes who are overweight and not on insulin (and therefore not at risk of going low overnight).

PERFECT PORTIONS

- *For many adults, eating 3–5 servings of carbohydrates at each meal and 1–2 servings of carbohydrates for each snack works well.*

- *Try to pair foods from different food groups together to reap the most nutritional benefits.*

- *For better portion control, serve your food on a 9-inch (23-cm) plate. At most meals, aim to fill half the plate with non-starchy vegetables, one-quarter of the plate with protein, and one-quarter of the plate with starchy vegetables.*

Snacks and beverages

- Choose beverages like water, seltzer (soda water), and unsweetened tea and coffee instead of sweet drinks like sodas (carbonated drinks), juices, and sports and energy drinks.

- A glass or two of red wine is not forbidden; just keep in mind that you should never drink on an empty stomach because of the risk of hypoglycemia when the liver is occupied with breaking down the alcohol and not releasing glucose.

- Dextrose tablets are the best portable snacks—always make sure to carry some with you.

- Other great ideas for healthy snacks include apple slices with peanut butter, veggies and hummus, Greek yogurt with granola, or a sliced banana with almond butter.

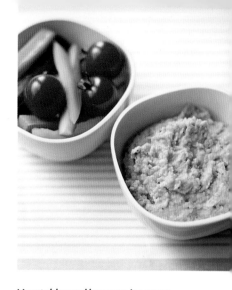

Vegetables and hummus is a great healthy snack—try the hummus recipe on page 127.

Special diets and diabetes

People with diabetes who need specific diets, other than just being careful about the carb content, must think carefully about their balance. Avoiding gluten is not necessarily good although many individuals with T1D also have gluten intolerance. Being a vegan or vegetarian can be positive, but often such diets are high in starch and thus carbs. Increasing the amount of leafy greens and veggies that are not starch based is a good thing, but make sure you get enough lean protein and some fats and long-acting carbs for the calorie content and to balance the sugar.

A low-carb diet

My attitude toward nutrition is pretty stringent. I do not like adding unnecessary calories and carbs to my system, which have been shown to not only lead to weight gain, but also to increased sugar values, higher needs for insulin, and thus greater risk for hypoglycemia. Higher blood sugars for a sustained period of time have been shown to increase risks for late-stage complications such as kidney, eye, and heart disease, and recently there is research linking cognitive dysfunction to high sugars and even Alzheimer's disease.

When a person with diabetes restricts carbs, the need for medications, including insulin, is diminished. The pancreas (in T2D) does not have to produce as much insulin, and there is less sugar converted into fat, leading to the added benefit of a leaner body. All the recipes in this book take this fact into account, only adding carbs as grains and fruits, rather than processed sugars. The addition of sugar to any food is not necessary, and I avoid it even with my new transplanted pancreas. I also avoid pasta, potatoes, and white rice, since these foods are high in simple carbs; I don't feel the need to add them for taste or calories.

Changes in dietary advice for diabetics

It is interesting to see how the attitude toward nutrition has changed over the years, despite more and more knowledge about the dangers of sugars and simple carbs. When I was diagnosed in 1989, the majority of T1D people were thin or average weight, while T2D were almost always overweight unless they took their disease seriously and changed behavior to avoid the progression toward insulin dependence. My initial therapy was the Novo pen, using two kinds of human insulin—basal insulin (long-acting) injected once a day and short-acting insulin before each meal. I had to time my meals carefully, since the insulin was less fast-acting than nowadays, and the long-acting insulin didn't completely cover me for twenty-four hours.

If diagnosed today, I would have been recommended an insulin pump, or so-called continuous insulin therapy, which, as it sounds, provides a basal rate of insulin throughout the day, and only requires dialing up the delivery of insulin when or prior to eating carbs. This therapy, together with improved glucose measuring tools, such as continuous glucometers worn on the abdomen and small, sophisticated episodic meters that measure the blood glucose in five seconds, has given people with diabetes much more freedom as well as better control.

However, the other big change compared to twenty-five years ago is the approach healthcare professionals and people involved in the diabetes infrastructure have taken when it comes to living life with diabetes, including restricting diet and limiting dosing. I was told to never touch toast, pancakes, soft drinks, or other foods containing very high carbs that did not bring nutrition. I was educated by dieticians who explained the effects of the toasted surface of a piece of bread versus a piece of bread that was made out of multigrain and not toasted. I was recommended not to drink orange juice or eat potatoes, and definitely not have cinnamon buns, a very common treat in my home country of Sweden. Today, we are learning more and more about the risks of sugar on our health, as related to heart disease, Alzheimer's, and obesity, and people all over the world are trying low-carb approaches to lose or maintain weight as well as improve cognitive functions and reduce morbidities.

Eating "normally" vs. a healthier lifestyle

Today, we are seeing a surprising phenomenon in the T1D community. There is an inherent conflict between the T1D and T2D camps, with some from the former almost discriminating against the latter, and not wanting to learn from or be mixed up with each other. Parents of T1D children and people living with T1D see themselves as having a disease that they did not deserve, while they see the disease T2D as a sign of laziness and lack of discipline. The truth remains that as T2D progresses, people with that type of diabetes end up with a poorly functioning pancreas, and will need to use the same kind of

Eating healthy meals, such as the Mediterranean Fattoush with Chicken on page 78, can be a joy rather than a punishment.

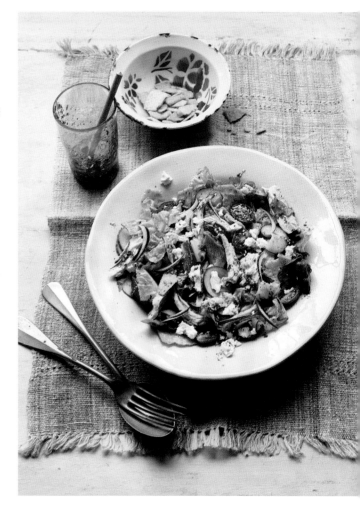

approach to therapy as the T1D crowd. The complicating problem in the case of T2D is the initial manifestation and the very cause of the disease, insulin resistance.

Going back to the late 1980s and early 1990s, when I was a young person with diabetes and new to this, I was presented with some advice and comments that surely are not used any longer—I was told that having diabetes would give me a head start on a healthy approach to life and that there were certain signs that I could learn to observe and act upon. At sixteen, and a serious athlete, I was eating a lot to fuel my body, but anyone going through puberty and reducing the amount of activity due to increasing demands from school risks weight gain. I was educated about the diet that would keep my sugars stable and that happens to be a kind of diet that is good for everyone. I realized I would have to say no to certain treats and foods, and that my friends and uninformed colleagues would look at me a little differently unless I opened up about the reasons to be diligent about sugar and simple carbs, but most of the time I saw it as an opportunity to stay healthy, not just with my diabetes, but with my weight, my body, and my mind.

I have to admit that there were a number of occasions when I heard people asking about me, and even confronting me about my restrictions, and it was awkward because I was very secretive about my T1D, but I did not care. In contrast, what I am seeing now is that parents and people with T1D are more concerned about "being allowed to eat normally" and "enjoying treats," as long as one dials up the pump and measures the blood glucose often. I am not against diligent control and being on top of one's measurements—this is critical and has really become easier with today's technology—but what I find sad is that people with T1D are supposedly not changing behavior to accommodate their disease and even more importantly, taking advantage of their disease to live a healthy life.

Double diabetes is increasing dramatically, and what it means is that one suffers from both T1D and T2D, by having T1D and then eating the wrong foods, dialing up the insulin, increasing in weight, and then becoming insulin resistant. Insulin is a metabolic factor, allowing for glucose to be used for energy by the cells including the brain, but it is also an anabolic hormone that builds fat when in excess. As a person with T1D I used about 2–6 units of insulin prior to my meals, and nowadays it is not unusual for people to be using ten times that amount due to insulin resistance. People with this condition are not only at increased risk of microvascular complications if they do not exert glucose control, but they also have increased risk of cardiovascular disease and orthopedic conditions due to their bodies being overweight and their insulin resistance.

I do not want us to go back to old technology and I do not want to discriminate against people with diabetes when it comes to their diets, but I urge parents and people with diabetes to consider their diagnosis as an opportunity to live a healthier lifestyle than if they had not been diagnosed. Healthy food can be and is delicious. There is no advantage to letting your child enjoy frosted birthday cakes or drinking cola. In fact, if one starts early, children do not get addicted to the high-sugar meals that will get them into so much trouble later on. I am not prescribing diet plans that are boring and resemble health spa visits, but there are a number of ways to provide healthy meals that will possibly convert other parents into treating their kids to a so-called "diabetic" diet.

! REMEMBER

- Preventing, reversing, and maintaining control of T2D is possible if implementing a stringent low-carb diet.

- Weight control is important in all types of diabetes, since weight increase leads to insulin resistance, and worse overall outcomes.

- Your insulin requirements are directly related to your diet and thus it is critical to understand the impact of food on your sugar values, for both people on insulin and people who are not on insulin.

- Excessive insulin dosing or increased endogenous (the body's own) insulin production lead to weight gain and further need for more insulin.

- A low-carb diet does not have to be boring, since there are many delicious food items that have plenty of healthy fats and proteins.

BREAKFAST RECIPES

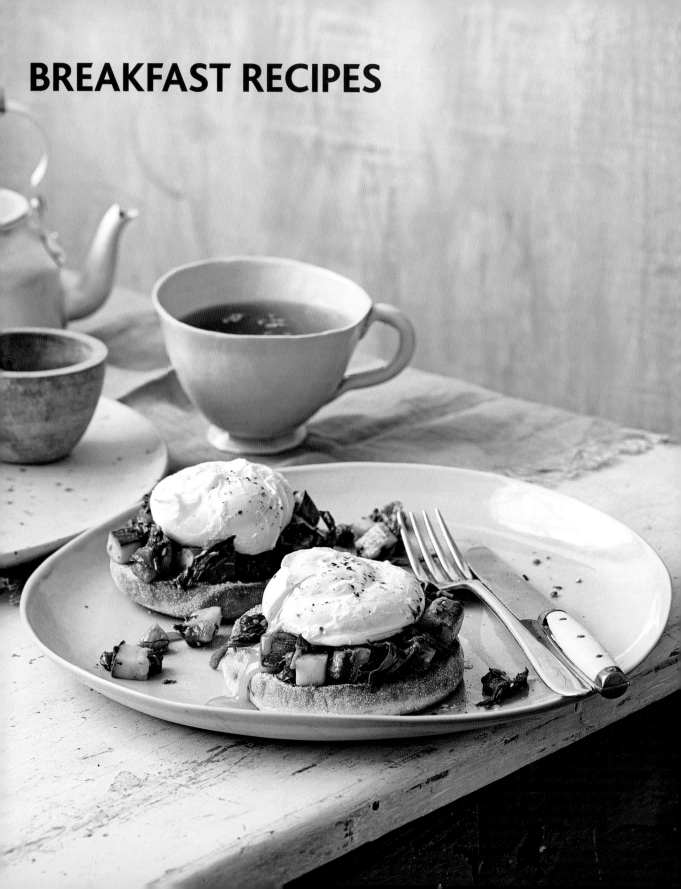

Vegetarian Eggs Benedict

2 tablespoons extra virgin olive oil

1 zucchini (courgette), diced

1 tomato, diced

1 cup (160 g) frozen chopped spinach

1/4 cup (25 g) pitted black olives, sliced

1/2 teaspoon dried rosemary

4 eggs

2 gluten-free English muffins, split in half

Salt and freshly ground black pepper

Serves 2

This hearty vegetarian dish will provide you with ample protein and carbohydrates to help you make it through the morning. If you're not sensitive to dairy, you can also add mozzarella cheese as a topping.

1 Heat the oil in a sauté pan over medium heat. Add the zucchini (courgette), tomato, spinach, olives, and rosemary, lightly season with salt and pepper, and sauté for about 5 minutes until the zucchini and tomato are softened and the spinach is heated through.

2 Meanwhile, poach the eggs. Fill a skillet (frying pan) with water and bring the water to a low boil. Break the eggs directly into the simmering water and cook for about 4 minutes until the yolk is as you desire.

3 While the eggs are poaching, toast the muffins in a toaster.

4 To assemble, place two muffin halves on each plate and top each muffin half with some sautéed vegetables and a poached egg.

Per serving: 489 kcals, 27.7 g fat (1.2 g saturates), 30.3 g carbohydrate (6.9 g sugars), 25.1 g protein, 7.4 g fiber, 2.2 g salt

Egg "Muffins"

Butter, for greasing

6 slices (rashers) of thin bacon

6 eggs

1 tablespoon heavy (double) cream

3 tablespoons chopped fresh herbs, such as oregano, rosemary, or basil

Salt and freshly ground black pepper

Makes 6 muffins

These filling and satisfying "muffins" are delicious. They taste great when served at room temperature, which makes them ideal for a quick breakfast, a snack, or to bring along for a picnic.

1 Preheat the oven to 400°F/200°C/Gas 6 and grease a 6-cup muffin pan with butter.

2 Use a slice (rasher) of bacon to line the inside each muffin cup.

3 Whisk together the eggs and cream in a bowl. Stir in the herbs and season with salt and pepper. Pour the egg mixture evenly into the prepared muffin cups.

4 Bake the muffins in the preheated oven for 15–20 minutes until the eggs are cooked and the muffins have a golden tone. Let cool for a few minutes before serving. The muffins will keep for 2–3 days in an airtight container in the refrigerator.

Tip: For a more filling dish, try adding some leftover cooked vegetables to the egg mixture.

Per muffin: 133 kcals, 10.5 g fat (3.8 g saturates), trace carbohydrate (trace sugars), 9.6 g protein, trace fiber, 0.7 g salt

Scrambled Quinoa

2 eggs

Pinch of salt

1 teaspoon butter (or coconut oil), for frying

½ cup (90 g) cooked quinoa

1 cup (about 75–100 g) leftover cooked or fresh vegetables, such as cauliflower, broccoli, asparagus, green beans, bell peppers, or leafy greens

Pinch of red pepper flakes

Serves 1

I always have some cooked quinoa on hand so that I can make this dish. Cooked and cooled quinoa will keep for 3–5 days in an airtight container in the refrigerator.

1 In a small bowl, whisk together the eggs with the salt.

2 Melt the butter or oil in a nonstick skillet (frying pan) over medium heat. Reduce the heat to low, then pour the eggs into the skillet, as if you were making scrambled eggs, and add the quinoa, vegetables, and red pepper flakes. Gently stir together all the ingredients until the eggs are cooked through.

Per serving: 286 kcals, 13.1 g fat (3.5 g saturates), 19.1 g carbohydrate (4.2 g sugars), 20.5 g protein, 4 g fiber, 1 g salt

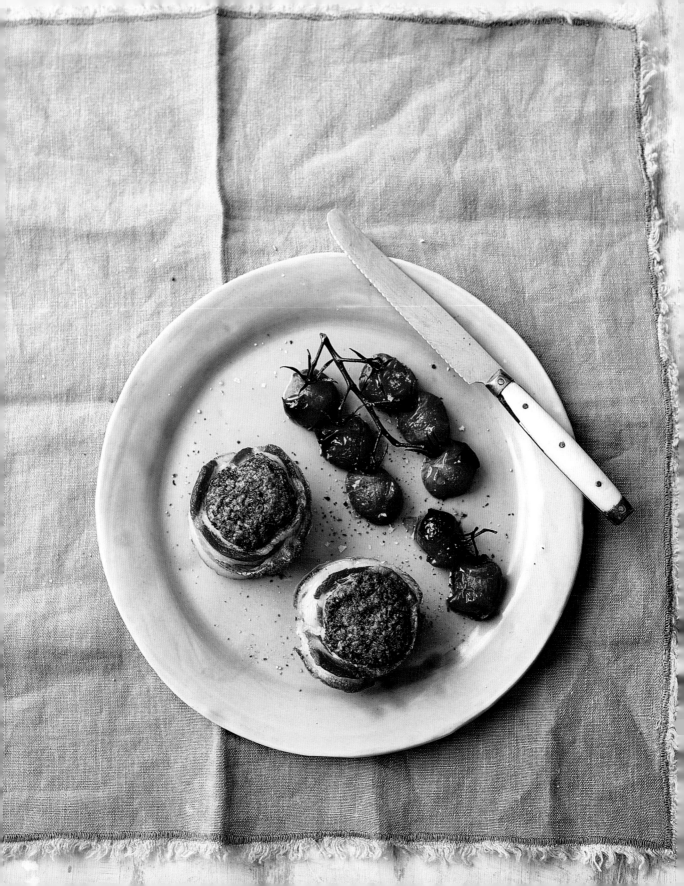

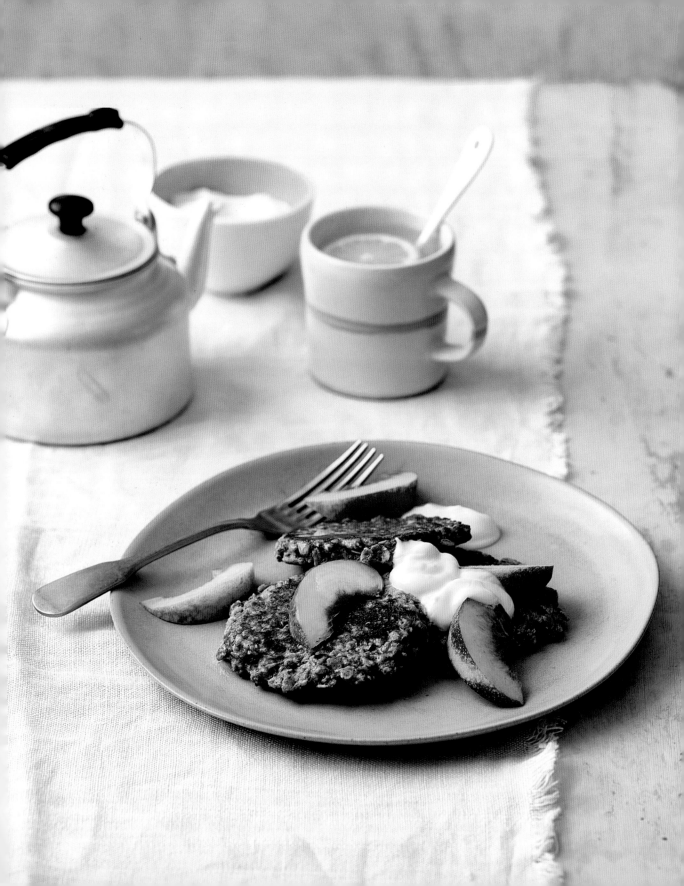

Pr-OAT-ein Pancakes

These simple pancakes (pictured left) are made mostly from egg and oats, creating a high-protein healthy breakfast option that won't weigh you down with too many refined carbohydrates.

1 First, make the batter. Mix together the oats, egg or egg whites, baking powder, vanilla extract, cinnamon, and banana or pumpkin purée in a bowl. Let sit for at least 5 minutes, or make the batter the night before and leave in the refrigerator.

2 Melt the butter or oil in a nonstick skillet (frying pan) over a medium heat. Pour the batter into the skillet to form two disk-shaped pancakes and cook for 2–3 minutes on each side until golden brown on both sides. Serve immediately, topped with nut or seed butter, yogurt, or fruit.

Per serving: 265 kcals, 9.5 g fat (2.8 g saturates), 29.9 g carbohydrate (9.4g sugars), 12.6 g protein, 4 g fiber, 0.9 g salt

$^1/_3$ cup (30 g) rolled or quick oats

1 large (medium) egg, or $^1/_3$ cup (75 ml) egg whites (from about 1–2 eggs)

$^1/_2$ teaspoon baking powder

$^1/_2$ teaspoon vanilla extract

$^1/_4$ teaspoon ground cinnamon

$^1/_2$ banana, mashed or 2 tablespoons pumpkin purée (optional)

$^1/_4$ teaspoon butter or oil, for frying

Serves 1

Cinnamon Pecan Oatmeal

Try this recipe instead of buying packaged oatmeal that typically contains excessive amounts of added sugars. The peanut butter, pecans, and flaxseeds provide protein and heart-healthy fats and the oats supply fiber in this nutrient-dense dish.

4 cups (950 ml) water

$^1/_3$ cup (40 g) chopped pecans

2 cups (275 g) steel-cut (coarse) oats

1 tablespoon unsweetened peanut butter

2 tablespoons ground flaxseeds

$^1/_2$ teaspoon ground cinnamon

$^1/_2$ teaspoon ground nutmeg

$^1/_4$ teaspoon salt

About $^1/_4$ cup (60 ml) unsweetened almond or soy milk

Serves 4

1 Pour the water into a saucepan and bring to a rolling boil. Slowly stir the pecans and oats into the boiling water, then stir in the peanut butter and cook for 5 minutes. Reduce the heat and simmer for 10–15 minutes, until the oats are soft in texture.

2 Add the flaxseeds, cinnamon, nutmeg, and salt, then slowly stir in the milk until the oatmeal is your desired consistency—you may not need to add all the milk. Serve hot.

Per serving: 394 kcals, 16 g fat (2.3 g saturates), 45 g carbohydrate (1.5 g sugars), 11.2 g protein, 9.6 g fiber, 0.4 g salt

Berry "Butter" Drizzle Bowl

1 tablespoon almond butter

1/2 tablespoon melted coconut oil

1 cup (125 g) fresh berries, such as a mixture of blueberries, chopped strawberries, and raspberries

1/2 tablespoon hemp seeds

1/2 tablespoon cocoa nibs

Serves 1

One cup of fresh berries counts as a serving of carbohydrate. Mixing almond butter with melted coconut oil creates a drippy drizzle that tastes like an ice cream topping, but is much healthier (pictured right). The coconut oil is delicious but a little high in saturates, so try to eat meals lower in saturated fats for the rest of the day.

1 To make the drizzle, mix together the almond butter and coconut oil in a small bowl.

2 Pile the berries into a bowl, sprinkle the hemp seeds and cocoa nibs over the top, then pour over the drizzle.

Per serving: 342 kcals, 25.8 g fat (9.5 g saturates), 10.5 g carbohydrate (7.3 g sugars), 9.1 g protein, 13.1 g fiber, 0.3 g salt

Salmon and Dill Frittata

1 x 7 1/2-oz (213-g) can salmon (choose a variety without oil or salt), drained

1/2 teaspoon salt

2 teaspoons lemon juice

1 tablespoon chopped fresh dill (or 1/2 teaspoon each dried oregano and dried basil)

2 eggs

1 teaspoon butter or extra virgin olive oil

Freshly ground black pepper

Serves 2

This frittata is the ideal choice for a light lunch or hearty breakfast. Serve it with whole grain bread for breakfast or a mixed green salad for lunch. The recipe scales up well, and the frittata tastes good when served cold too.

1 Preheat the broiler (grill) to medium–high.

2 Put the salmon in a bowl and mash it with a fork to break up all the flesh, skin, and bones. Stir in the salt, lemon juice, and dill, season with pepper, and mix well with the fork. Add the eggs and mix in thoroughly.

3 Heat the butter or oil in an ovenproof skillet (frying pan) over medium heat until bubbling. Add the salmon mixture and use a rubber spatula to distribute it evenly in the skillet. Reduce the heat to low and cook for 5–6 minutes until the sides are set—the whole frittata should slide around when you shake the skillet.

4 Place the skillet under the preheated broiler (grill) and cook for 3 minutes, or until the frittata is cooked through and golden. Slide the frittata onto a large plate or chopping board, cut in half, and serve immediately.

Per serving: 257 kcals, 14.3 g fat (4.1 g saturates), 0.1 g carbohydrates (0.1 g sugars), 31.9 g protein, trace fiber, 1.5 g salt

Avocado Smoothie

Avocados contain fiber, healthy unsaturated fats, and a variety of helpful micronutrients. Consider giving your smoothie a nutritional boost by adding a tablespoon of ground flaxseeds for additional fiber and omega fatty acids.

1 ripe avocado, peeled and stoned

2 cups (475 ml) unsweetened almond milk

2 scoops (60 g) whey protein

½ cup (70 g) crushed ice

Serves 2

1 Combine all the ingredients in a food processor or blender and blend until smooth.

2 Pour the smoothie into 2 glasses and serve immediately.

Per serving: 332 kcals, 20.7 g fat (4.2 g saturates), 7.5 g carbohydrate (3 g sugars), 27 g protein, 4.9 g fiber, 0.5 g salt

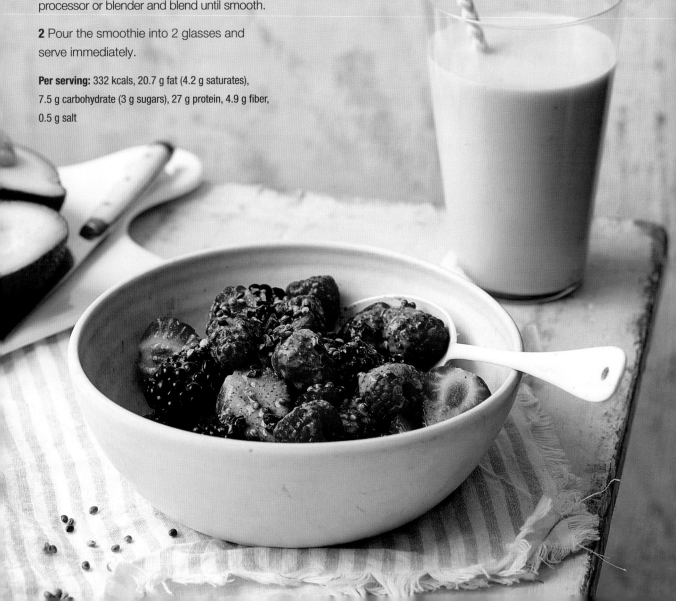

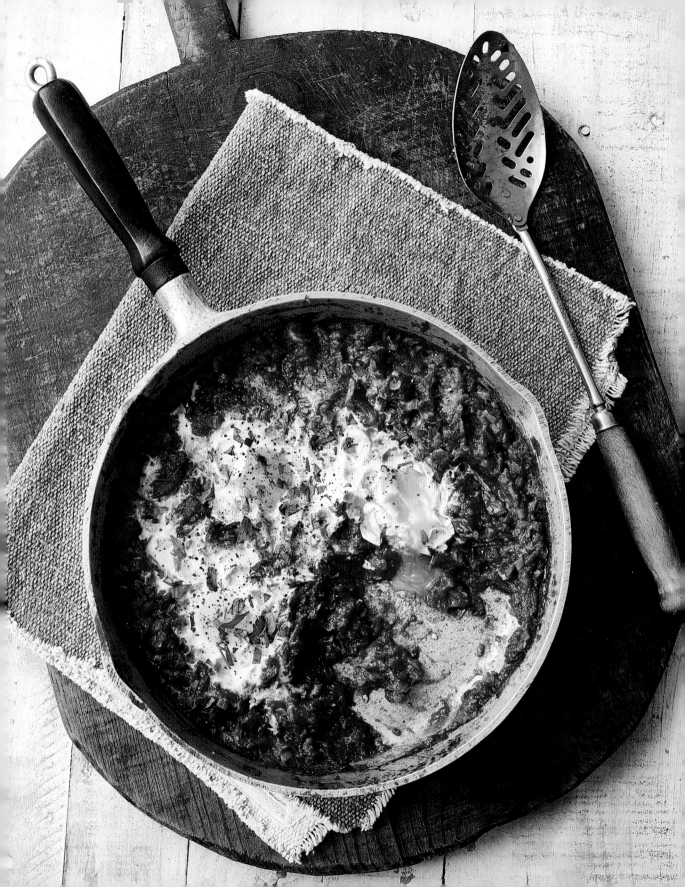

It's the Weekend Shakshuka

2 tablespoons olive oil

1 small yellow onion, finely chopped

2 garlic cloves, minced

1 green or red bell pepper, seeded and finely chopped

1 teaspoon paprika

1/2 teaspoon ground cumin

1 x 28-oz can (2 x 400-g cans) diced tomatoes (or 4 cups/650 g diced fresh tomatoes)

1 tablespoon tomato paste (purée)

4–6 large (medium) eggs

Salt and freshly ground black pepper

1/2 cup (10 g) chopped fresh herbs, such as mint, flat-leaf parsley, cilantro (coriander), or basil, to garnish (optional)

Whole wheat pita bread, to serve

Serves 4

Here is a great weekend breakfast that combines brightly-colored vegetables with eggs for a Mediterranean-style meal. The eggs cook right in the tomato sauce, so this is a one-pan meal.

1 Heat the oil in a large skillet (frying pan) with a lid over medium heat, add the onion and garlic, and cook for about 5 minutes, stirring occasionally, until soft and starting to brown. Add the bell pepper, paprika, and cumin and sauté for 3–5 minutes, then add the tomatoes and tomato paste (purée) and simmer for an additional 3–5 minutes until the tomatoes are warmed through and the sauce just starts to bubble.

2 Make 4–6 small divots in the sauce and carefully crack an egg into each divot. Cover and simmer for 10–15 minutes, until the eggs are cooked and the sauce is slightly reduced. Season with salt and pepper and garnish with fresh herbs, if using. Scoop the shakshuka onto 4 plates, and serve with whole wheat pita bread.

Per serving: 288 kcals, 19.3 g fat (3.5 g saturates), 11.8 g carbohydrate (11.2 g sugars), 14.7 g protein, 3.4 g fiber, 0.6 g salt

Cottage Cheese and Avocado Toast

Half a cup of low-fat cottage cheese contains almost 15 grams of protein with less than 5 grams of carbohydrate. There is no need to add extra salt as the cottage cheese is already salty.

2 slices whole wheat bread

1/2 small avocado or 1/4 large avocado, sliced

1/2 cup (115 g) low-fat cottage cheese

Freshly ground black pepper

Serves 1

1 Preheat the broiler (grill) to medium–high. Toast the slices of bread under the broiler (grill).

2 Place the toast on a plate. Arrange the avocado slices on the toast, then spoon the cottage cheese on top, and finish with a generous grinding of pepper.

Per serving: 387 kcals, 17.4 g fat (4.7 g saturates), 33.6 g carbohydrate (6 g sugars), 20.3 g protein, 8.5 g fiber, 1.4 g salt

LIGHT MEALS and SALADS

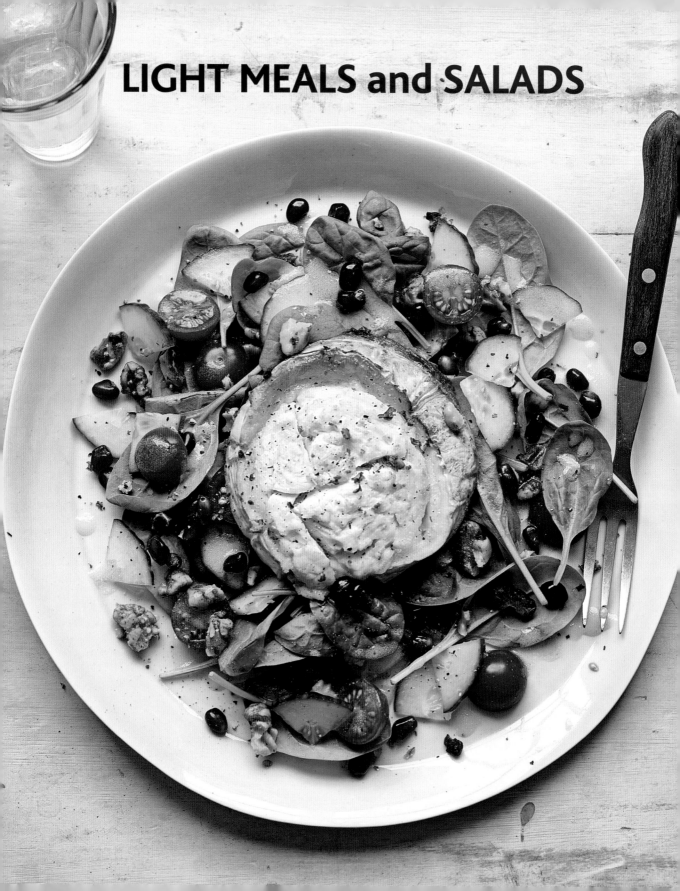

Goat Cheese Salad

4 slices of chèvre (goat cheese), about 1½ oz (45 g) each

2¼ cups (100 g) baby leaf spinach

15 cherry tomatoes, halved

1 cucumber, chopped

A handful of chopped walnuts or seeds (you could try pumpkin, sunflower, or flax seeds)

Seeds of 1 pomegranate

FOR THE DRESSING

3½ tablespoons (50 ml) olive oil, plus extra for greasing

3 tablespoons white vinegar

1 teaspoon Dijon mustard

Pinch of salt

Pinch of freshly ground black pepper

Serves 4

This fresh summer salad combines all the good things in life. Goat cheese is made out of goats' milk, and is ideal if you can't tolerate lactose. Goat cheese is often used in French cuisine and has a characteristic flavor that is a joy for the taste buds.

1 Preheat the oven to 400°F/200°C/Gas 6 and grease a baking sheet with oil.

2 Put the chèvre slices on the prepared baking sheet and bake in the preheated oven for 15 minutes, or until the edges of the chèvre slices are bubbling and brown.

3 Meanwhile, in a large bowl, mix together the spinach, tomatoes, and cucumber.

4 Heat a dry nonstick skillet (frying pan) over medium heat, add the walnuts or seeds and toast, stirring frequently, until golden brown. Add the walnuts or seeds to the salad.

5 Make the dressing by whisking together the oil, vinegar, mustard, salt, and pepper in a small bowl.

6 Divide the salad among plates, top each with a slice of the warm goat cheese, sprinkle the pomegranate seeds over the top, and drizzle with the dressing.

Per serving: 348 kcals, 28 g fat (10.1 g saturates), 8.2 g carbohydrate (8 g sugars), 13.7 g protein, 3.5 g fiber, 1 g salt

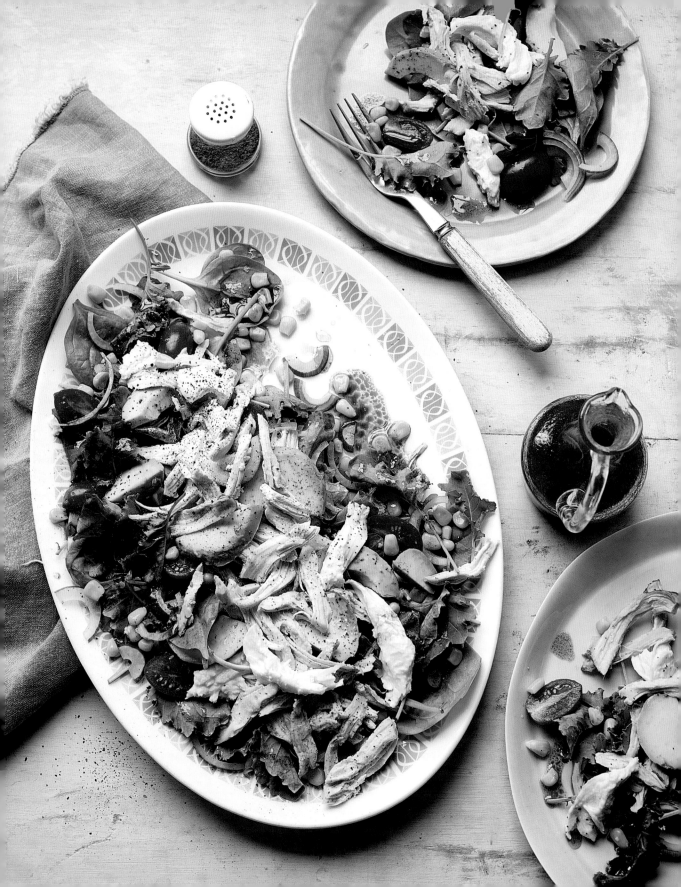

Chicken, Avocado, and Tomato Salad

Consuming enough vegetables throughout the day can be difficult, especially when salads are often the side event at the dinner table. This low-carb salad provides everything needed to serve as a main course, and can be used as a foundation to add more of your favorite vegetables to your diet.

1 Toss the spinach, kale, onion, tomatoes, corn, and vinaigrette together in a salad bowl. Let sit for 5 minutes at room temperature.

2 Arrange the chicken, avocado, and mozzarella on top of the salad and serve immediately.

Per serving: 441 kcals, 23.6 g fat (7.8 g saturates), 15 g carbohydrate (8 g sugars), 45 g protein, 6.4 g fiber, 0.8g salt

3¹/₂ cups (150 g) baby leaf spinach

3¹/₂ cups (150 g) baby kale

¹/₂ small red onion, cut into ¹/₄–¹/₂-inch (5-mm–1-cm) slices

¹/₂ cup (85 g) cherry tomatoes, halved or whole

¹/₄ cup (70 g) frozen corn, thawed

¹/₂ cup (120 ml) balsamic vinaigrette

8 oz (225 g) cooked chicken breast, shredded

¹/₂ ripe avocado, peeled, stoned, and cut into ¹/₄–¹/₂-inch (5-mm–1-cm) slices

2¹/₄ oz (60 g) sliced mozzarella cheese

Serves 2

Zucchini, Walnut, and Lemon Salad

¹/₂ cup (50 g) chopped walnuts

3 zucchini (courgettes), very thinly sliced lengthwise

¹/₄ cup (5 g) coarsely chopped fresh flat-leaf parsley

FOR THE DRESSING

4 tablespoons olive oil

Grated zest and juice of 1 unwaxed lemon

2 pinches of salt

Pinch of freshly ground black pepper

Serves 4 as a side dish, 2 as a main meal

This appetizing salad makes a great side dish for a barbecue, or you can enjoy it on its own as a light and refreshing meal.

1 Heat a dry skillet (frying pan) over medium–high heat, add the walnuts, and toast, stirring frequently, until golden brown.

2 In a small bowl, whisk together the oil, lemon zest and juice, salt, and pepper to make a dressing.

3 Put the zucchini (courgettes), walnuts, and parsley in a salad bowl, pour over the dressing, and mix thoroughly.

Per serving (if serves 4): 292 kcals, 27.4 g fat (3.2 g saturates), 4 g carbohydrate (3.7 g sugars), 5.3 g protein, 3.5 g fiber, 0.3 g salt

Tuna Melt Tartines

1 x 5-oz (160-g) can tuna in water, drained

2 celery stalks, finely diced

2 tablespoons finely diced red onion

1 small apple, cored and finely diced

1 teaspoon Dijon mustard

1 tablespoon Greek yogurt

Pinch of salt

Pinch of freshly ground black pepper

4 slices whole grain or pumpernickel bread

2 x 1-oz (25-g) slices Cheddar cheese, torn in half

Serves 2

Pump up your tuna salad with celery, red onion, and diced apple, and use Greek yogurt instead of mayonnaise as it contains less saturated fat and will add extra protein to the dish. You can make these tartines with either whole grain or pumpernickel bread. The pumpernickel tastes particularly delicious with the Cheddar.

1 Preheat the oven to 450°F/230°C/Gas 8. Line a baking sheet with parchment (baking) paper or foil.

2 In a large bowl, mix together the tuna, celery, onion, apple, mustard, yogurt, salt, and pepper.

3 Place the slices of bread on the prepared baking sheet and divide the tuna salad among the 4 slices of bread. Top each tartine with half a slice of cheese. Bake in the preheated oven for 4–5 minutes until the cheese just melts.

Per serving: 441 kcals, 14.3 g fat (7.6 g saturates), 41 g carbohydrate (11.3 g sugars), 33.1 g protein, 7.2 g fiber, 2 g salt

Three Bean Salad

Beans are an excellent source of protein and fiber. This simple salad provides a meatless option for those who are vegetarian or looking to add a meat-free meal into their diet.

1 First make the dressing. Whisk together the oil, mustard, and garlic in small bowl. Set aside.

2 Put the beans, tomato, shallots or onions, bell pepper, and vinegar in a large bowl and toss well. Add the dressing and the parsley, then season with salt and pepper and gently stir all the ingredients together. Serve the salad cold or at room temperature.

Per serving: 274 kcals, 5.5 g fat (0.8 g saturates), 34.6 g carbohydrate (7.5 g sugars), 13.4 g protein, 13.4 g fiber, 2 g salt

8 oz (225 g) canned cannellini beans, rinsed and drained

8 oz (225 g) canned black beans, rinsed and drained

8 oz (225 g) canned kidney beans, rinsed and drained

1 large tomato, cut into $1/2$-inch (1-cm) cubes

$1/8$ cup (15 g) minced shallots or onions

$1/2$ cup (90 g) chopped green bell pepper

$1/4$ cup (60 ml) balsamic vinegar

3 tablespoons finely chopped curly parsley

Salt and freshly ground black pepper

FOR THE DRESSING

1 tablespoon olive oil

2 tablespoons Dijon mustard

2 tablespoons minced garlic

Serves 4

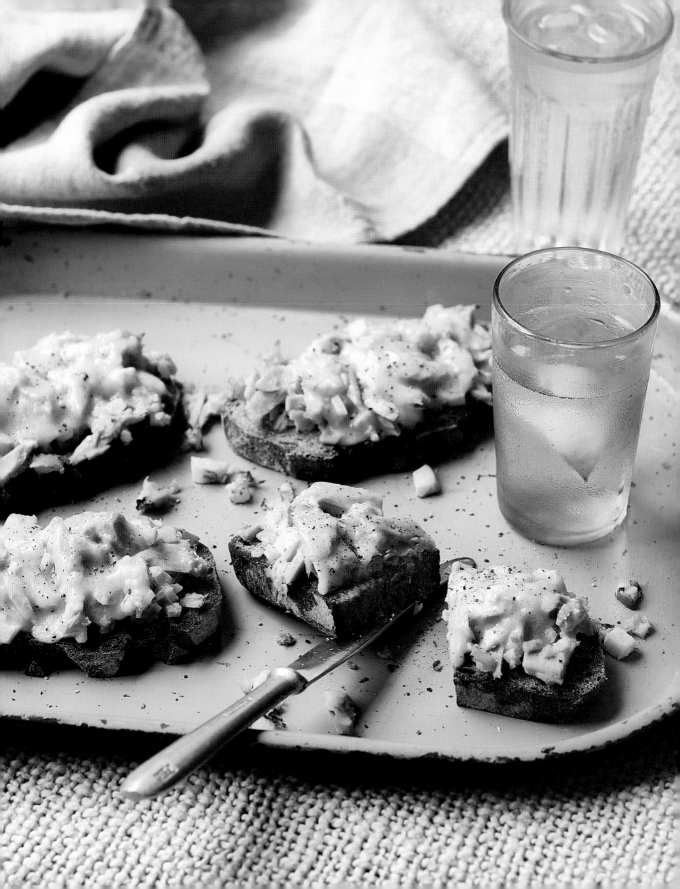

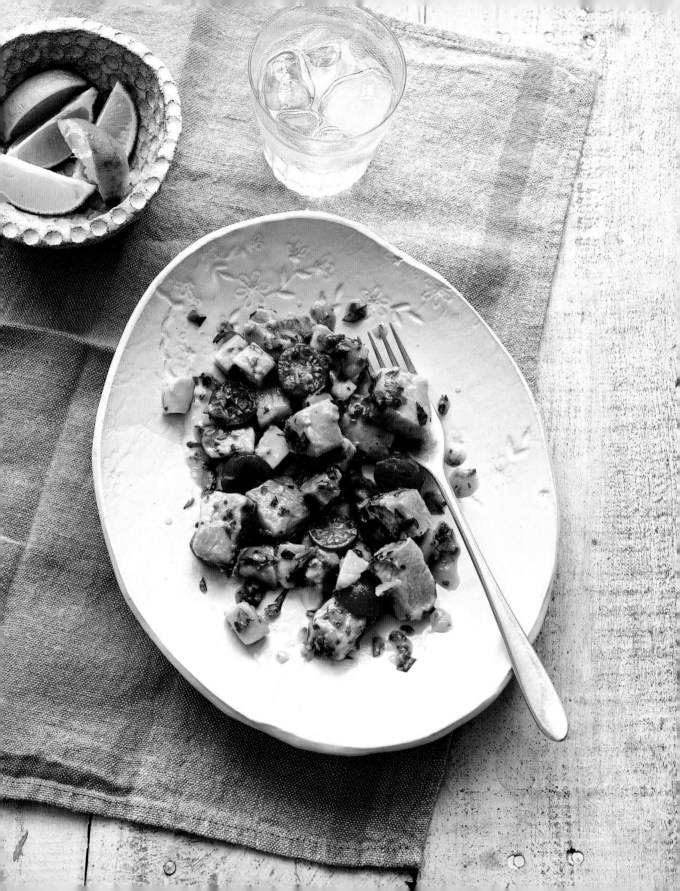

Salmon Ceviche

This wonderfully refreshing dish can be served as an appetizer or a main course. Sashimi-grade salmon is frozen right after being caught in order to kill any parasites before the fish is consumed raw. Sashimi- (or sushi-) grade means that it is the highest quality fish on offer in a store.

1 Put all the ingredients in a nonmetallic bowl and mix together.

2 Cover with plastic wrap (clingfilm) and place in the refrigerator for at least 2 hours.

Per serving (if serves 4): 244 kcals, 20.7 g fat (3.7 g saturates), 2 g carbohydrate (1.5 g sugars), 11.4 g protein, 1.8 g fiber, 0.1 g salt

7 oz (200 g) sashimi-grade raw salmon, cut into bite-sized pieces

1 avocado, peeled, stoned and chopped

5 cocktail tomatoes, halved

Juice of 2 limes

2 tablespoons olive oil

A handful of chopped fresh cilantro (coriander)

2 small chiles, seeded and chopped

Serves 4 as an appetizer, 2 as a main meal

Bowtie Pasta and Tuna Salad

This recipe combines two favorites—tuna salad and pasta salad—into one. The addition of broccoli, pine nuts, and olive oil and the use of whole wheat pasta make this salad high in fiber and heart-healthy unsaturated fats.

4 garlic cloves, minced

1 small onion, cut into $1/2$-inch (1-cm) cubes

$1/3$ cup (20 g) broccoli florets (the florets should be about 1 inch/2.5 cm in size)

2 tablespoons olive oil

$1/4$ cup (60 ml) water

$1^1/3$ cups (85 g) whole wheat bowtie (farfalle) pasta

1 x 12-oz can (3 x 120-g cans) tuna, drained

$1/3$ cup (50 g) crumbled feta cheese

2 tablespoons pine nuts

$1^1/2$ tablespoons chopped fresh basil

$1/4$ teaspoon salt

$1/2$ teaspoon freshly ground black pepper

Serves 4

1 Preheat the oven to 400°F/200°C/Gas 6.

2 Place the garlic, onion, and broccoli in an ovenproof dish and pour the oil over the vegetables. Add just enough water to cover the bottom of the dish to a depth of about $1/4$ inch (5 mm). Cover and bake in the preheated oven for 40 minutes, or until the vegetables are soft.

3 Meanwhile, bring a large pan of water to a boil and cook the pasta according to the package directions. Drain well.

4 To assemble the salad, put the baked vegetables, pasta, tuna, feta, pine nuts, basil, salt, and pepper in a large bowl and gently mix together. Serve the salad warm or cold.

Per serving: 277 kcals, 13.5 g fat (3.1 g saturates), 15.5 g carbohydrate (2.2 g sugars), 21.3 g protein, 3.4 g fiber, 0.7 g salt

Mediterranean Fattoush with Chicken

This salad essentially follows the principles of the Plate Method, which helps people plan balanced meals. It contains non-starchy vegetables, protein from the chicken and the cheese, and starch from the pita chips. Making your own salad dressing is easy, and the end result tends to be lower in sodium and free of preservatives as compared to store-bought dressings. Za'atar is a Mediterranean spice that can be found in most grocery stores. If you cannot find it, try mixing together ¼ teaspoon of ground cumin and ½ teaspoon of sesame seeds instead.

1 Combine all of the salad ingredients in a large bowl.

2 Whisk together the oil, lemon juice, and za'atar in a small bowl. Toss the dressing with the salad.

Per serving: 504 kcals, 28 g fat (6.6 g saturates), 19.1 g carbohydrate (12.4 g sugars), 34.7 g protein, 6.2 g fiber, 1.2 g salt

FOR THE SALAD

1 head lettuce, chopped into bite-sized pieces

½ red onion, thinly sliced

1 heaped cup (170 g) cherry or grape tomatoes, halved

½ large cucumber, thinly sliced into rounds

⅓ cup (50 g) feta cheese, crumbled

1 cup (150 g) cubed cooked chicken breast

1 cup (60 g) pita chips

FOR THE DRESSING

2 tablespoons olive oil

1½ tablespoons lemon juice

½ teaspoon za'atar

Serves 2

Toasted Chicken Sandwich

When choosing whole wheat bread, always check the ingredients and select the one with 100 percent whole wheat as the first ingredient. Also, read the label and choose a bread with about ½ oz (15 g) of total carbohydrates per serving. This sandwich can also be made with untoasted bread.

5–6 oz (150–175 g) cooked chicken breast, cut into ½-inch (1-cm) slices

1 teaspoon balsamic vinaigrette

2 slices whole wheat bread

½ cup (20 g) baby leaf spinach or baby kale

1 tomato, cut into ¼-inch (5-mm) slices

Serves 1

1 Put the chicken and vinaigrette in a small bowl and toss together until the chicken is completely coated with the vinaigrette.

2 Toast the bread in a toaster.

3 To assemble the sandwich, place a slice of toast on a plate, arrange the chicken on top, followed by the spinach or kale and tomato, and then finish with the second slice of toast.

Per serving: 445 kcals, 6.4 g fat (1.4 g saturates), 35.5 g carbohydrate (6.9 g sugars), 57 g protein, 7.7 g fiber, 1.1 g salt

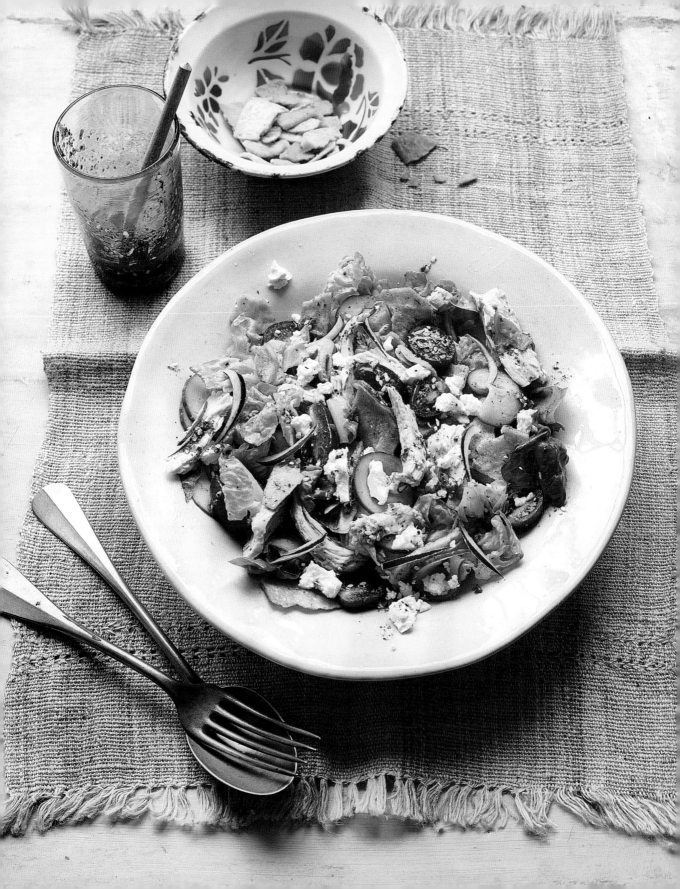

MAIN MEALS

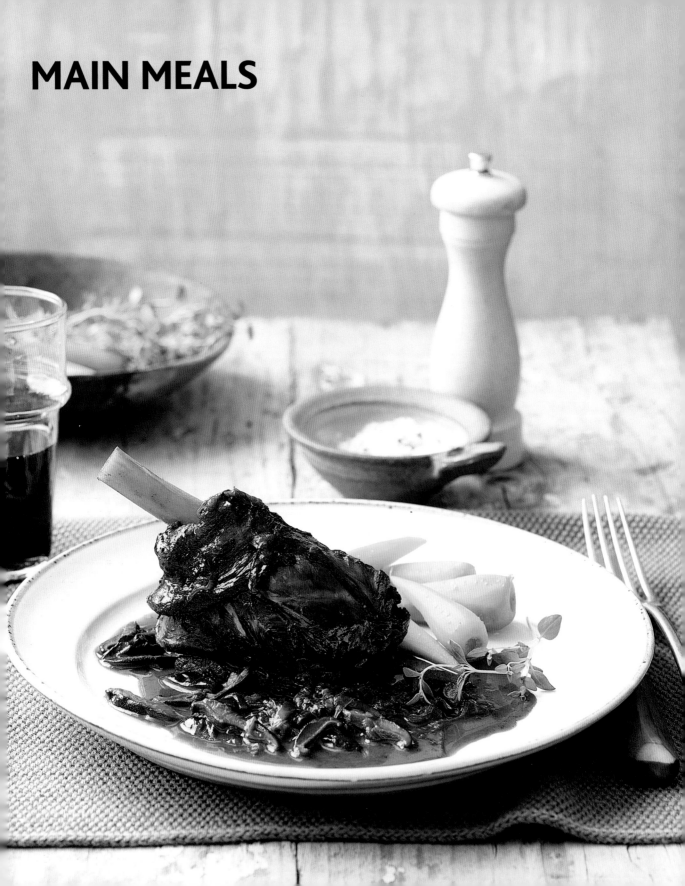

Braised Lamb Shanks with Shiitake Mushrooms

4 lamb shanks

Unbleached white flour, for dusting

2 tablespoons extra virgin olive oil

2 onions, thinly sliced

4 garlic cloves, thinly sliced

1 cup (250 ml) red wine

3 cups (750 ml) chicken stock

10 fresh thyme sprigs, plus extra to garnish

8 oz (225 g) fresh shiitake mushrooms, stems removed and caps thinly sliced

Salt and freshly ground black pepper

1¹/₂ lb (675 g) cooked carrots, to serve

Serves 4

These braised lamb shanks cook largely unattended for 2 hours, until the meat is falling off the bone. This dish tastes even more delicious if it is made a day in advance; and if you do this you can also skim off any fat that collects on the top of the sauce.

1 Preheat the oven to 325°F/160°C/Gas 3.

2 Season the lamb shanks with salt and pepper. Spread out the flour on a plate. Put the lamb shanks on the plate and turn over until coated in the flour.

3 Heat the oil in a large Dutch oven (casserole dish) over medium–high heat. Add the lamb shanks and sauté for 3–4 minutes on all sides until golden.

4 Transfer the lamb shanks to a plate and then pour off all but a couple of tablespoons of fat from the Dutch oven. Reduce the heat to medium, add the onions and garlic, and stir to scrape up any brown bits from the bottom of the pan, then sauté for about 10 minutes until softened. Add the wine and cook until reduced by half, about 5 minutes. Add the stock, thyme, and mushrooms, return the lamb shanks to the Dutch oven, and bring to a boil.

5 Cover and place in the preheated oven for 2 hours, or until the meat is falling off the bones. Turn the oven temperature up to 500°F/260°C/Gas 10 and cook, uncovered, for an additional 20 minutes, basting frequently, until the lamb shanks are well browned. Remove from the oven.

6 Using a slotted spoon, transfer the lamb shanks to a plate. Place the Dutch oven on the stove over high heat and cook for about 10 minutes, until the juices have reduced and thickened. Remove and discard the thyme sprigs (most of the leaves will have fallen into the pot). Skim off any fat with a bulb baster or slotted spoon. Taste the sauce and season with salt if necessary. Return the lamb shanks to the sauce in the Dutch oven. Serve with cooked carrots and garnish with fresh thyme.

Tip: If you're sensitive to gluten or have hypothyroidism, use gluten-free flour.

Per serving: 687 kcals, 38.1 g fat (14.7 g saturates), 23.3 g carbohydrate (16.3 g sugars), 50 g protein, 8.3 g fiber, 1.7 g salt

Chana Masala

1 tablespoon canola (rapeseed) oil

2 onions, finely diced

1 garlic clove, minced

2 teaspoons grated fresh ginger

2 teaspoons ground coriander

$1/2$ teaspoon cayenne pepper

1 teaspoon ground turmeric

2 teaspoons ground cumin

2 teaspoons paprika

1 teaspoon garam masala

$1/2$ teaspoon ground cinnamon

2 cups (325 g) chopped fresh tomatoes or 1 x 15-oz (400-g) can whole tomatoes with their juices, chopped

$2/3$ cup (150 ml) water

2 x 15-oz (400-g) cans chickpeas, drained and rinsed

Pinch of salt

Juice of $1/2$ lemon

Serves 4–6

Try to make some of your meals vegetarian as this is a heart-healthy and environmentally-friendly way to eat. This Indian-inspired meal is full of fragrant spices. The chickpeas contain carbohydrates, but they also contain fiber and protein, making them a "complex carbohydrate."

1 Heat the oil in a large skillet (frying pan) over medium–high heat. Add the onions, garlic, and ginger and sauté until starting to brown, about 5 minutes.

2 Turn the heat down to medium, add the coriander, cayenne, turmeric, cumin, paprika, garam masala, and cinnamon, and cook for another minute. Add the tomatoes and their juices, followed by the water and chickpeas. Simmer for about 10 minutes to let the flavors meld, then add the salt and lemon juice. Serve the chana masala with cooked brown rice, quinoa, or couscous.

Per serving (if serves 4): 217 kcals, 4.7 g fat (0.4 g saturates), 28.2 g carbohydrate (9.2 g sugars), 10 g protein, 9.2 g fiber, 0.4 g salt

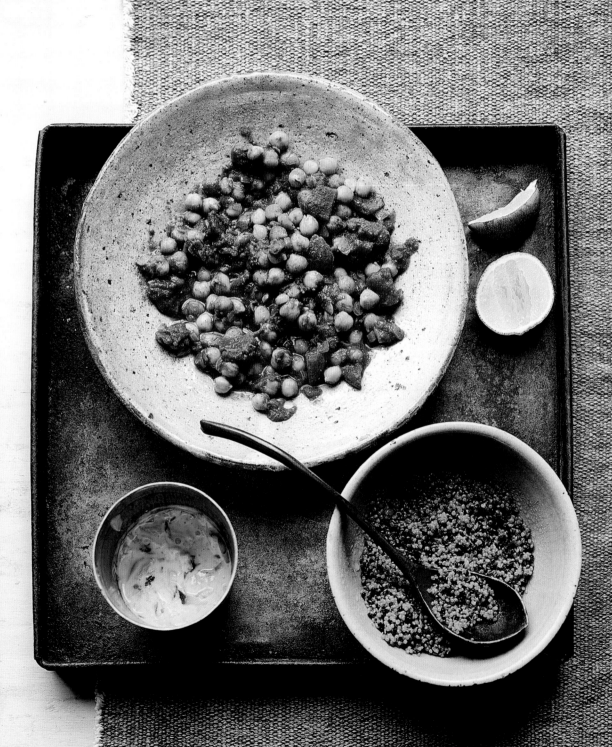

Chinese Tilapia Hot Pot

At Chinese Lunar New Year, and on many other occasions, families in China and Taiwan gather around a simmering pot of broth at the table and share treasures of the sea and land poached right at the table. Once the fish has been eaten, the final step is to turn the simmering broth into noodle soup. If the pot can be kept over a Sterno (canned heat) or portable burner, that's great. If not just make sure the broth is boiling hot when it gets to the table, and then reheat it before adding the noodles. Tilapia is one of the most sustainable, eco-friendly fish available.

1 First make the dipping sauce. Whisk together the shoyu or tamari (soy sauce), sugar, and oil in a small bowl. Divide this sauce among four dipping bowls.

2 Set a Sterno (canned heat), portable burner, or trivet in the middle of the dining table, and put out a soup plate and a portion of dipping sauce at each place setting, along with soup spoons and chopsticks or forks.

3 In a saucepan that is large enough to hold all ingredients, combine the water, stock, daikon radish, and mushrooms. Bring to a boil, then reduce the heat and simmer for 15 minutes. Add the fish, shrimp (prawns), and vegetables and bring back to a simmer, then immediately transfer the saucepan to the Sterno, portable burner, or trivet on the dining table.

4 Place a slotted spoon in the saucepan and allow your guests to help themselves to portions of fish, shrimp, and vegetables. Guests dip their items in their dipping sauce as they eat.

5 Once the fish is gone, bring the stock back to a boil, add the noodles, and simmer for 5 minutes. Spoon the noodles and broth into the soup bowls to serve.

Tip: For a heartier meal, you could add 8 oz (225 g) Chinese dumplings (or 1 lb/450 g stuffed Chinese dumplings) to the saucepan with the noodles and simmer for 5 minutes.

Per serving: 211 kcals, 5.5 g fat (0.9 g saturates), 10.7 g carbohydrate (3.9 g sugars), 28.7 g protein, 2.6 g fiber, 4.8 g salt

4 cups (950 ml) water

4 cups (950 ml) low-sodium chicken stock

2-inch (5-cm) piece of daikon radish, cut into chunks

1/2 cup (15 g) dried mushrooms, such as shiitake, soaked in a bowl of hot water for 15 minutes, then drained and cut into slices

1 lb (450 g) tilapia fillet, sliced into 1/2-inch (1-cm) strips

12 raw shrimp (prawns), peeled and deveined

8 oz (225 g) Asian green vegetables, such as baby bok choy or water spinach (available in Asian grocery stores), cut into pieces if large

1 x 1-oz (25-g) bundle bean thread noodles (sometimes called glass or cellophane noodles, available in Asian grocery stores), soaked in a bowl of warm water for 15 minutes, then drained

FOR THE DIPPING SAUCE

1/2 cup (120 ml) reduced-salt shoyu or tamari (soy sauce)

1/4 teaspoon Sucanat (a brand of whole cane sugar), coconut sugar, or honey

1 tablespoon toasted sesame oil

Serves 4

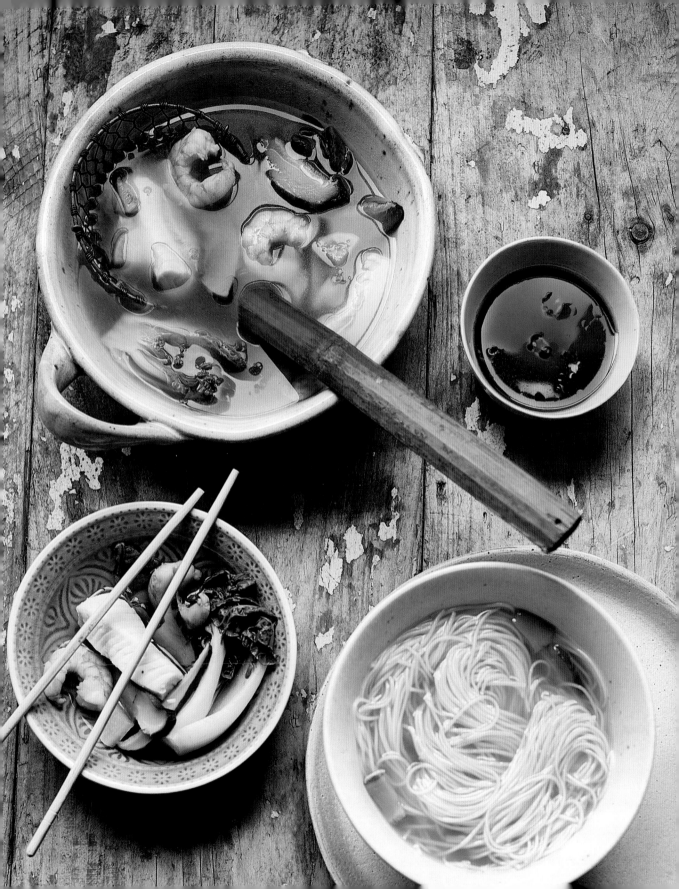

Flounder with Zucchini, Tomatoes, and Oregano

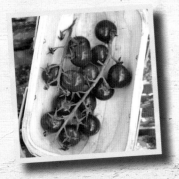

Flounder laid on top of a bed of caramelized zucchini (courgette) and cherry tomatoes takes on great flavor and cooks quickly. I've used dried oregano and fresh thyme, but feel free to improvise with rosemary, parsley, or whatever herbs you have on hand.

2 teaspoons extra virgin olive oil, coconut oil, or ghee

1 small zucchini (courgette), halved lengthwise and thinly sliced into half-moons

1 cup (170 g) cherry tomatoes, halved

Pinch of dried oregano

2 flounder fillets or other flatfish, about 4–6 oz (120–175 g) each

1 teaspoon fresh thyme leaves (optional)

A few drops of freshly squeezed lemon juice

Salt and freshly ground black pepper

Serves 2

1 Heat the oil or ghee in a large skillet (frying pan) over medium–high heat. Add the zucchini (courgette) and a sprinkling of salt and pepper and cook for about 3 minutes, turning the slices a couple of times, until most of the slices are golden.

2 Reduce the heat to medium-low and add the tomatoes and oregano. Layer the fish on top of the vegetables and sprinkle with salt and pepper and the thyme, if using. Cover and cook for 5 minutes, or until the flounder is cooked through.

3 Transfer the fish to two plates and top with the vegetables. Sprinkle some lemon juice over the top and serve hot.

Per serving: 197 kcals, 7.6 g fat (1.3 g saturates), 4.1 g carbohydrate (4.1 g sugars), 26.7 g protein, 2.3 g fiber, 0.6 g salt

Barley, Lamb, and Swiss Chard Soup

1 lb (450 g) boneless lamb shoulder, trimmed and cut into 1-inch (2.5-cm) pieces

1 tablespoon extra virgin olive oil

2 onions, cut into small dice

3 celery stalks, cut into small dice

3 carrots, chopped

8 cups (1.9 liters) reduced-salt vegetable stock

2 bay leaves

1 small fresh rosemary sprig

¾ cup (140 g) pearl barley, rinsed and drained

4 Swiss chard leaves, stems removed and leaves cut into ½-inch (1-cm) ribbons

Salt and freshly ground black pepper

Serves 8

Lamb and barley are a happy pairing but as a one-pot meal they can be too heavy. The addition of chard creates a lighter dish and provides a nice textural addition.

1 Season the lamb with salt and pepper.

2 Heat the oil in a Dutch oven (casserole dish) over medium–high heat. Add the lamb and cook until it is browned on all sides, about 5 minutes. Remove from the heat and use a slotted spoon to transfer the lamb to a clean bowl.

3 Place the Dutch oven back on the stove, add the onions, celery, carrots, and ½ teaspoon of salt, and cook over medium heat for 5 minutes, or until the vegetables are slightly softened. Add the stock, bay leaves, and rosemary, return the lamb to the Dutch oven, and bring to a simmer, stirring to scrape up any brown bits from the bottom of the Dutch oven.

4 Reduce the heat to a medium and simmer for 30 minutes, or until the lamb is tender. Stir in the barley and simmer for a further 30 minutes, or until the barley is completely tender. Turn off the heat.

5 Remove and discard the bay leaves and rosemary. Stir in the chard and let stand for about 5 minutes until it has wilted. Season to taste with salt and pepper.

Per serving: 247 kcals, 10.2 g fat (3.9 g saturates), 23.5 g carbohydrate (8.2 g sugars), 13.7 g protein, 4.1 g fiber, 1.5 g salt

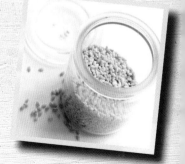

2 x 3-oz (80-g) packs ramen noodles, the flavor packet discarded

1/4 cup (60 g) peanut butter

1 tablespoon soy sauce

1 tablespoon rice vinegar

1/2 red bell pepper, thinly sliced into strips

1/2 yellow or orange bell pepper, thinly sliced into strips

1 carrot, sliced into matchsticks

Serves 2

Ramen Noodles with Peanut Sauce and Peppers

Ramen gets an upgrade with a comforting peanut sauce and raw veggies. Toss out the flavor packet that comes with the ramen noodles, as it contains salt and preservatives.

1 Bring a large saucepan of water to a boil. Once boiling, add the ramen noodles and cook for 2–3 minutes, or according to the package directions. Using tongs or a slotted spoon, take out the cooked noodles and transfer to a large bowl. Reserve the cooking water.

2 To make the peanut sauce, combine the peanut butter, soy sauce, and vinegar in a small bowl and whisk together—it will be very thick. Whisk in ¼ cup (60 ml) of the reserved cooking water to thin the sauce.

3 Add the peanut sauce, bell peppers, and carrot to the bowl with the cooked ramen noodles and toss well. Serve immediately.

Per serving: 514 kcals, 17.6 g fat (4.2 g saturates), 65 g carbohydrate (11 g sugars), 18.4 g protein, 9.3 g fiber, 2.5 g salt

---

3 teaspoons olive oil, divided

1 lb (450 g) ground (minced) chicken breast

1 teaspoon chopped fresh rosemary or thyme

Pinch of salt

Pinch of freshly ground black pepper

2½ cups (150 g) spinach, chopped

1 cup (175 g) couscous

Serves 6

Chicken and Spinach Couscous

This is a great weeknight dinner because everything cooks in 30 minutes or fewer. To make things even easier, use spinach that is already pre-washed.

1 Heat 2 teaspoons of the oil in a skillet (frying pan) with a lid over medium–high heat. Add the chicken, rosemary or thyme, salt, and pepper and sauté for about 5 minutes until the chicken is cooked. Add the spinach to the skillet with a splash of water. Cover and cook for 3–5 minutes until the spinach is just wilted.

2 Meanwhile, prepare the couscous according to the package directions.

3 Put the cooked couscous into the skillet with the chicken and spinach mixture, then add the remaining oil and toss well.

Per serving: 209 kcals, 3.8 g fat (0.7 g saturates), 19.7 g carbohydrate (0.4 g sugars), 22.2 g protein, 3 g fiber, 0.3 g salt

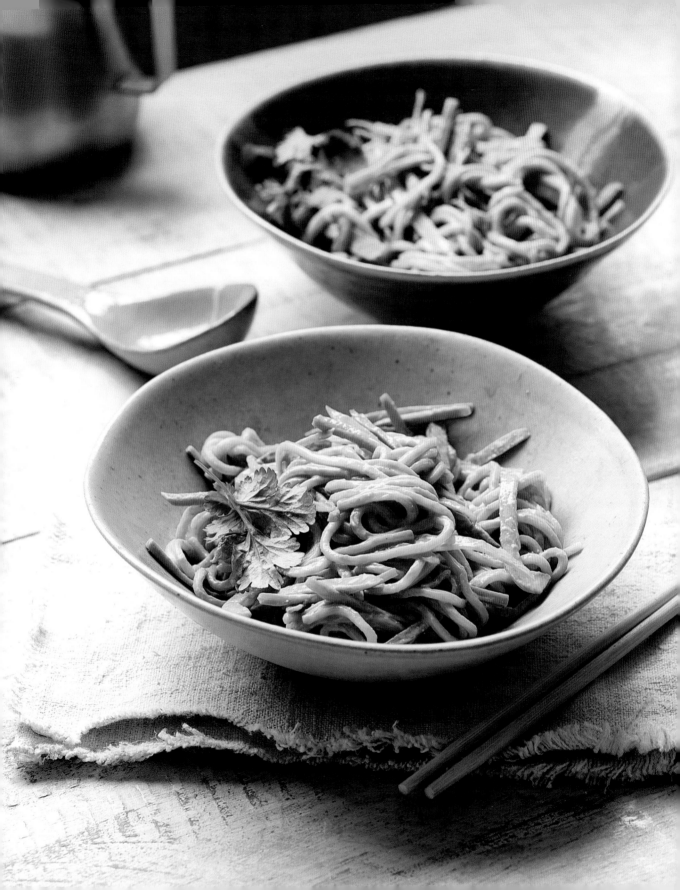

Classic Meatballs

Nonstick cooking spray, for greasing

8 oz (225 g) ground (minced) lean turkey

8 oz (225 g) ground (minced) pork

8 oz (225 g) ground (minced) extra-lean chicken

1¹⁄₂ tablespoons onion powder

1 tablespoon garlic powder

1 teaspoon freshly ground black pepper

1 lb (450 g) marinara sauce

2 tablespoons grated Parmesan cheese

TO SERVE

1 cup (135 g) cooked brown rice

1 large bunch of kale, steamed

Serves 3

Meatballs are often thought of as part of a larger pasta dish or as a filler for a meatball sub. This versatile and tasty low-fat meatball recipe can be served as a main meal with a balanced portion of steamed vegetables and brown rice or alone as a high-protein, no-carb snack.

1 Preheat the oven to 350°F/180°C/Gas 4. Grease a baking pan with nonstick cooking spray.

2 In a large bowl, mix together the ground (minced) meats, onion and garlic powders, salt, and pepper. Using your hands, shape the mixture into 12 meatballs —make sure they are all uniform in size to ensure they cook evenly.

3 Place the meatballs in the prepared baking pan and bake in the preheated oven until the meatballs reach an internal temperature of 165°F (75°C) on a meat thermometer, about 20–25 minutes. Transfer the meatballs to a plate and let rest for 5 minutes.

4 Meanwhile, 5 minutes before the end of the baking time for the meatballs, put the marinara sauce in a saucepan over medium heat and simmer the sauce for about 10 minutes, stirring occasionally. Season with salt and pepper.

5 To serve, divide the meatballs among bowls, pour over the marinara sauce, and sprinkle with the Parmesan. Serve with cooked brown rice and steamed kale.

Per serving: 534 kcals, 20.7 g fat (6.8 g saturates), 22.3 g carbohydrate (12.7 g sugars), 59 g protein, 6.1 g fiber, 1.8 g salt

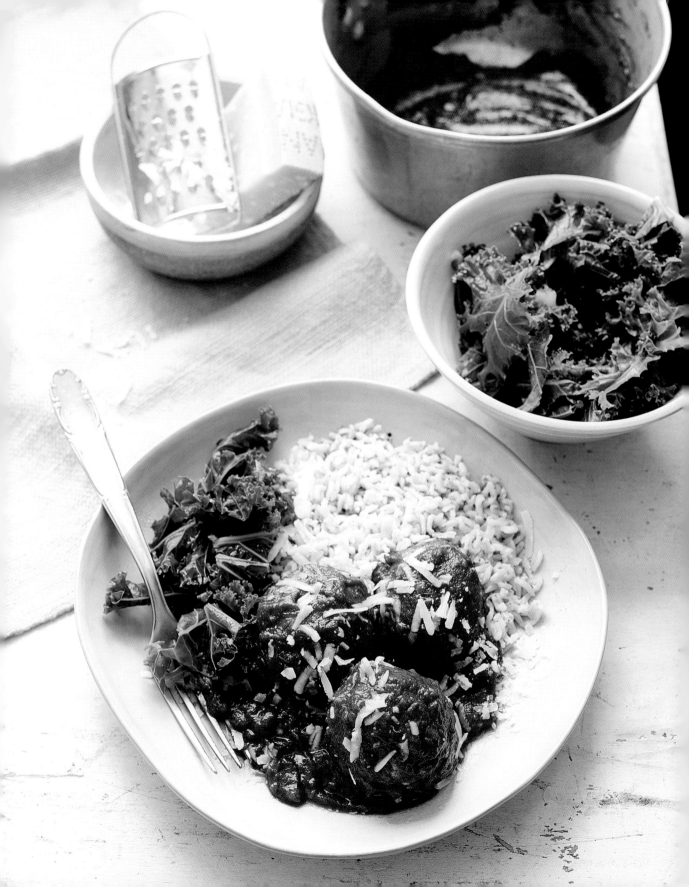

Chanterelle Mushroom and Stilton Quiche

FOR THE PIE CRUST

3 eggs

1 cup (110 g) coconut flour

1 tablespoon psyllium seed husks

1 teaspoon salt

7 tablespoons (100 g) melted butter, plus extra for greasing

FOR THE FILLING

2 tablespoons butter, for frying

3³⁄₄ cups (200 g) fresh chanterelle mushrooms

1 small onion, chopped (optional)

2 garlic cloves, crushed (optional)

¹⁄₂ cup (65 g) cubed Stilton cheese

¹⁄₂ cup (50 g) grated cheese (your favorite one)

3 eggs

³⁄₄ cup (200 ml) heavy (double) cream

Salt and freshly ground black pepper

FOR THE GREEN SALAD

2 cups (100 g) salad leaves, such as kale, romaine lettuce, Swiss chard, or spinach

1 cucumber, sliced

20 cherry tomatoes, halved

Serves 8

The pie crust for this flavorful low-carb quiche is made without wheat flour. Psyllium seed husks, an indigestible form of dietary fiber, are used to bind the crust ingredients together, in much the same way that gluten does in recipes containing wheat.

1 Preheat the oven to 350°F/180°C/Gas 4 and grease an 9-inch (23-cm) pie dish with butter.

2 To make the pie crust, put the eggs, coconut flour, psyllium seed husks, and salt in a large bowl and mix with a fork, then stir in the melted butter.

3 Tip the pie crust mixture into the prepared pie dish and press the mixture evenly into the bottom and sides of the dish. Bake in the preheated oven for about 8 minutes, or until the crust is golden.

4 Meanwhile, make the filling. Melt the butter in a skillet (frying pan), then add the mushrooms and the onion and garlic, if using, and cook over medium heat for 10 minutes, or until soft.

5 Spread the mushroom mixture over the crust base and then sprinkle the Stilton and grated cheese over the top.

6 Whisk together the eggs and heavy (double) cream in a bowl, season with salt and pepper, and then pour the cream mixture over the cheeses in the pie dish.

7 Turn the oven temperature down to 325°F/160°C/Gas 3. Place the pie dish in the oven and bake for 30 minutes, or until the filling has set.

8 Mix together the salad leaves, cucumber, and tomatoes in a salad bowl.

9 Serve the quiche immediately with the green salad.

Per serving: 435 kcals, 37.1 g fat (22.2 g saturates), 6.6 g carbohydrate (4.3 g saturates), 13.5 g protein, 8.6 g fiber, 1.6 g salt

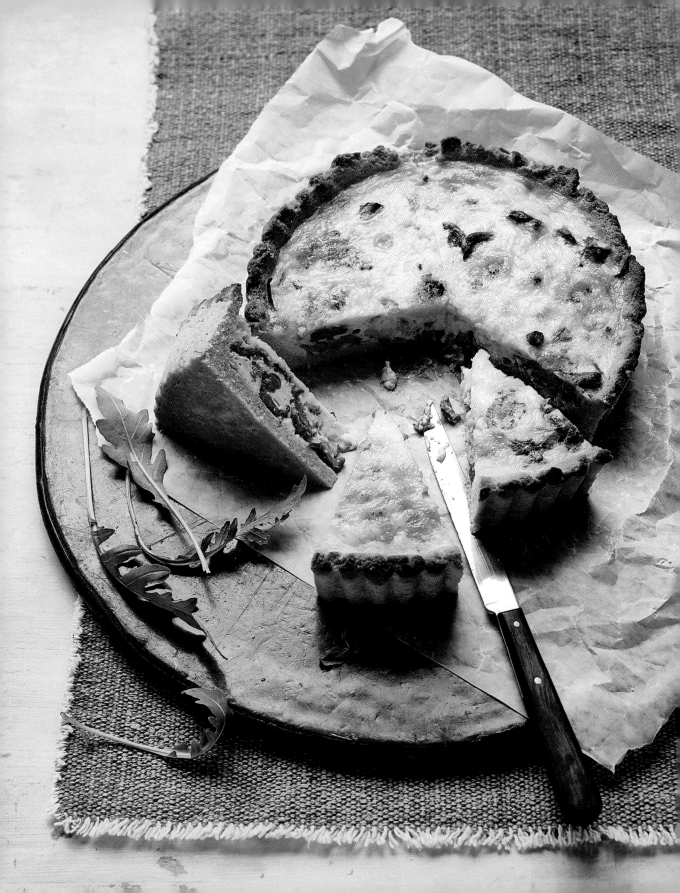

Teriyaki Steak Tips

2 lb (900 g) steak tips (or beef sirloin or fillet, cut into strips)

3/4 cup (175 ml) tamari (soy sauce)

1 3/4 cups (415 ml) water

1/2 cup (120 ml) apple cider vinegar

3 garlic cloves, minced

1-inch (2.5-cm) piece of fresh ginger, peeled and minced

1 teaspoon sesame seeds, for sprinkling

TO SERVE

3 cups (400 g) cooked brown rice

1 1/2 lb (675 g) steamed broccoli

Serves 6

If you're craving Chinese food but don't want all the salt and sugar found in many store-bought sauces, this is a tasty and healthy alternative.

1 In a large bowl, combine the steak tips, tamari (soy sauce), water, vinegar, garlic, and ginger. Cover with plastic wrap (clingfilm) and let marinate in the refrigerator for at least 2 hours, or preferably overnight.

2 About 1 hour before you are ready to cook, remove the bowl with the marinating steak from the refrigerator and let stand until it comes to room temperature.

3 Preheat the broiler (grill) to medium–high. Remove the steak tips from the marinade and place them on a broiler-proof (grill-proof) pan. Broil (grill) the steak tips for 7 minutes. Use tongs to flip the steak tips and continue cooking them for another 4–5 minutes until the thickest piece registers 145°F (63°C) on a meat thermometer.

4 Divide the steak tips among plates and sprinkle with the sesame seeds. Serve with cooked brown rice and broccoli.

Per serving: 370 kcals, 8.7 g fat (3.4 g saturates), 22.4 g carbohydrate (6.2 g sugars), 44 g protein, 5.2 g fiber, 1.2 g salt

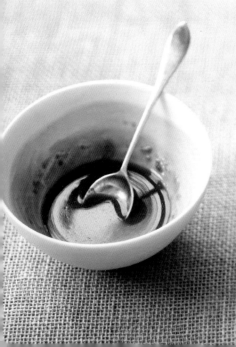

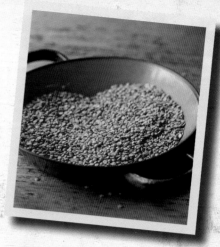

Vegan Lentil Soup

This hearty and filling meat-free soup is made with vegetables and lentils. The lentils provide an excellent source of protein and fiber.

3 tablespoons olive oil

1 onion, diced

2 tablespoons diced white mushrooms

3 garlic cloves, minced or crushed

¹⁄₃ cup (40 g) sliced carrots

¹⁄₂ teaspoon dried basil

¹⁄₂ teaspoon dried thyme

1 teaspoon salt

1 teaspoon freshly ground black pepper

6 cups (1.4 liters) water or vegetable stock

1 cup (165 g) lentils, rinsed and drained

1 x 28-oz can (2 x 400-g cans) diced tomatoes

1 teaspoon curry powder

2 teaspoons ground cumin

Juice of 1 small lemon

Serves 4

1 Heat the oil in a Dutch oven (casserole dish) over medium heat. Add the onion, mushrooms, garlic, carrots, basil, thyme, salt, and pepper and sauté until the onions are translucent.

2 Increase the heat to medium–high, add the water or vegetable stock, lentils, and tomatoes, and cook for 25–35 minutes, until the lentils and carrots are tender. Reduce the heat to medium, add the curry powder and cumin and cook for 15 minutes.

3 Remove from the heat and let sit for 5 minutes. Stir in the lemon juice and then serve.

Per serving (using water, not vegetable stock): 296 kcals, 10.8 g fat (1.5 g saturates), 33.7 g carbohydrate (11.8 g sugars), 13.2 g protein, 5.6 g fiber, 1.4 g salt

Chicken with Sun-dried Tomatoes, Olives, and Feta

4 boneless and skinless chicken breasts, about 4 oz (120 g) each

2 cups (200 g) pitted black or green olives

10 sun-dried tomatoes

1/3 cup (50 g) crumbled feta cheese

3/4 cup (200 ml) half and half (single) cream

FOR THE CAULIFLOWER MASH

1 head cauliflower, broken into florets and any tough stems cut off and discarded

2 tablespoons olive oil

Salt

Serves 4

A little Italian culinary flair is never a bad idea! This tasty dish can also be served with cooked vegetables or a salad.

1 Preheat the oven to 350°F/180°C/Gas 4.

2 Put the chicken breasts in a Dutch oven (casserole dish). Cover the chicken with the olives and sun-dried tomatoes, add the feta, then pour the cream over the top.

3 Bake in the preheated oven for 30–40 minutes until the chicken is cooked through.

4 Meanwhile, make the cauliflower mash. Bring a large saucepan of salted water to a boil. Add the cauliflower and cook for 10–15 minutes until tender. Remove the saucepan from the heat and drain any excess liquid. Use an immersion blender to purée the cauliflower, then stir in the olive oil, and process again until smooth.

5 Serve the chicken with the cauliflower mash.

Per serving: 338 kcals, 27.9 g fat (10.7 g saturates), 9.7 g carbohydrate (7.5 g sugars), 36.1 g protein, 5.3 g fiber, 2.4 g salt

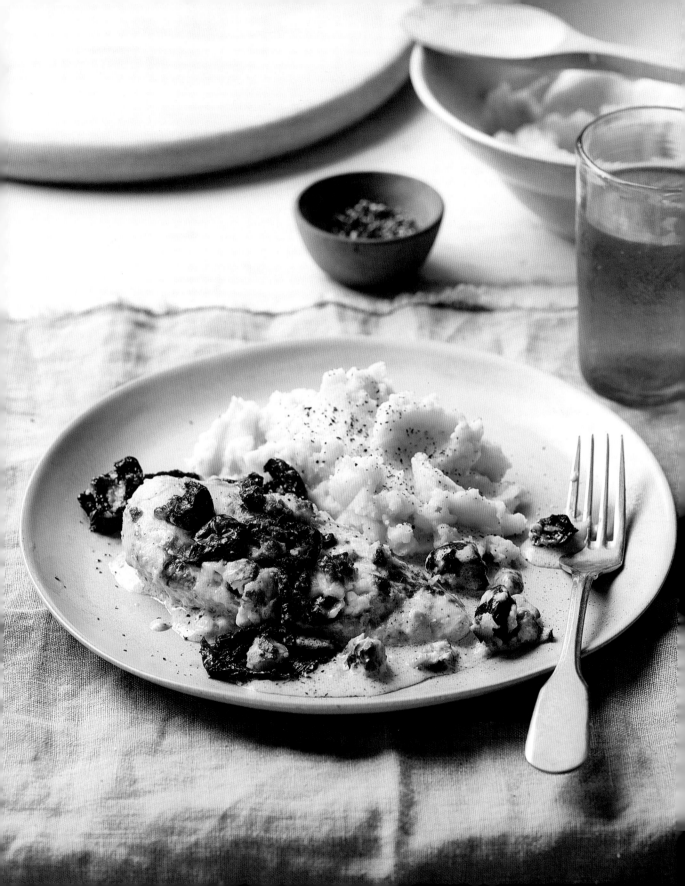

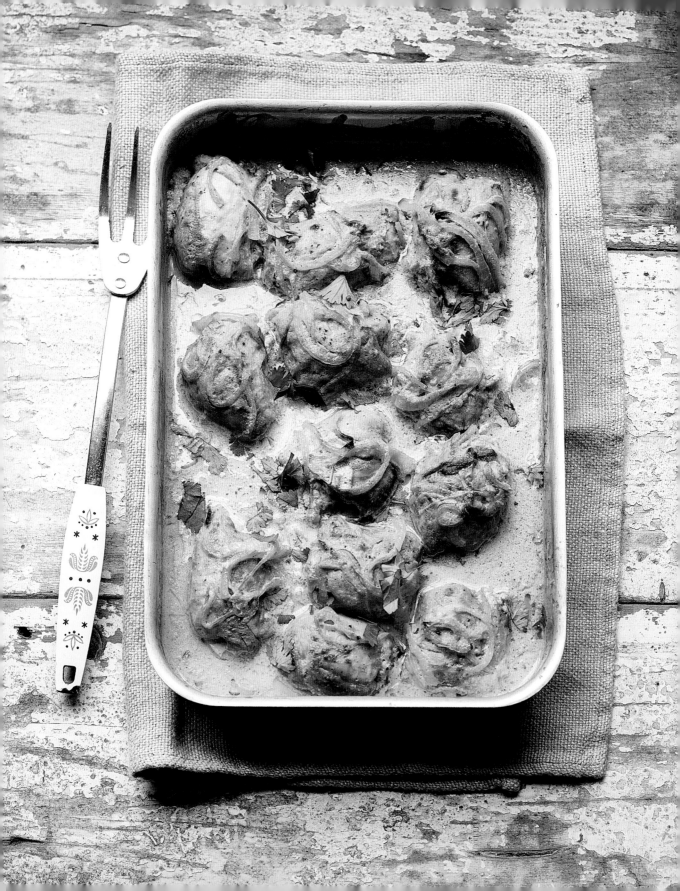

Baked Chicken with Curry Yogurt Sauce

2 lb (900 g) boneless and skinless chicken thighs

2 tablespoons extra virgin olive oil, divided

1 cup (130 g) sliced onions

2 garlic cloves, chopped

2 teaspoons curry powder

2 cups (430 ml) plain yogurt

Salt and freshly ground black pepper

TO SERVE

2 cups (250 g) cooked basmati or jasmine rice

1 cup (120 g) cooked peas, to serve

Serves 4

Succulent chicken thighs become extra exciting when paired with a simple and creamy curry sauce. Use your favorite curry powder and good-quality yogurt to make the recipe as piquant as you like and as satisfying as possible.

1 Preheat the oven to 425°F/220°C/Gas 7.

2 Place the chicken thighs in a baking pan and drizzle with 1 tablespoon of the oil. Rub the oil evenly over the chicken and sprinkle with a little salt and pepper. Bake in the preheated oven for 15 minutes.

3 Meanwhile, heat the remaining oil in a small saucepan over medium–low heat. Add the onions and cook for about 5 minutes, until slightly colored. Add the garlic and curry powder and cook for 2 minutes, then stir in the yogurt and heat through for a couple of minutes. Stir in ½ teaspoon of salt and a sprinkling of pepper.

4 Pour the yogurt sauce over the chicken. Cover with foil and continue to bake for an additional 15 minutes, until the chicken is cooked through and the juices run clear.

5 Mix together the cooked rice and peas and serve with the chicken.

Per serving: 596 kcals, 26.8 g fat (8.1 g saturates), 32 g carbohydrate (11.8 g sugars), 55 g protein, 3 g fiber, 0.9 g salt

White Fish Cakes with Dijon Dressing and Mixed Greens

8 cups (225 g) mixed greens, such as spinach, mesclun, lettuce, arugula (rocket), or any salad greens

Lemon wedges, to garnish

FOR THE DRESSING

1 shallot, coarsely chopped

2 tablespoons Dijon mustard

Juice of 1 lemon

1 tablespoon cold water

1/3 cup plus 1 tablespoon (100 ml) extra virgin olive oil

2 tablespoons finely chopped chives

FOR THE FISH CAKES

1 lb (450 g) cooked white fish, such as baked bass, steamed snapper, or broiled (grilled) tilapia

3/4 cup (40 g) breadcrumbs

1 egg, beaten

1/4 cup (5 g) flat-leaf parsley, chopped

2 teaspoons Dijon mustard

1 teaspoon Old Bay (or Cajun) seasoning

1 tablespoon extra virgin olive oil, for frying

Serves 4

A super-useful bit of leftover magic, this dish is the perfect way to utilize cooked fish of any kind. Of course, there's nothing wrong with cooking fish specifically for the cakes.

1 First make the dressing. Combine the shallot, mustard, lemon juice, and water in a food processor or blender and blend until smooth. With the motor running on high speed, gradually drizzle in the oil to form a creamy emulsified dressing. If the dressing is too thick you can thin it by adding a little extra cold water. Transfer to a bowl and stir in the chives.

2 Next, make the fish cakes. In a large bowl, gently fold together the fish, half of the breadcrumbs, egg, parsley, mustard, and Old Bay Seasoning, until the mixture forms a cohesive mass and can be formed into cakes. Using your hands, shape the mixture into 8 cakes, each about 1 inch (2.5 cm) thick.

3 Spread out the remaining breadcrumbs on a plate. Put the fish cakes on the plate and turn over until coated in the breadcrumbs.

4 Heat the oil in a large skillet (frying pan) over medium heat, and cook the fish cakes for 4 minutes on each side, until lightly browned.

5 In a large bowl, lightly toss the mixed greens with 2 teaspoons of the dressing.

6 Divide the salad among plates, arrange two fish cakes on top of each portion of salad, and dress liberally with remaining dressing. Serve garnished with lemon wedges.

Tips: If you have hypothyroidism, do not use spinach; instead, use other salad greens. If you have gout, use tilapia. Also, do not use spinach; instead, use other salad greens.

Per serving: 430 kcals, 28.3 g fat (4.1 g saturates), 6.8 g carbohydrate (2.1 g sugars), 32.8 g protein, 3 g fiber, 1.9 g salt

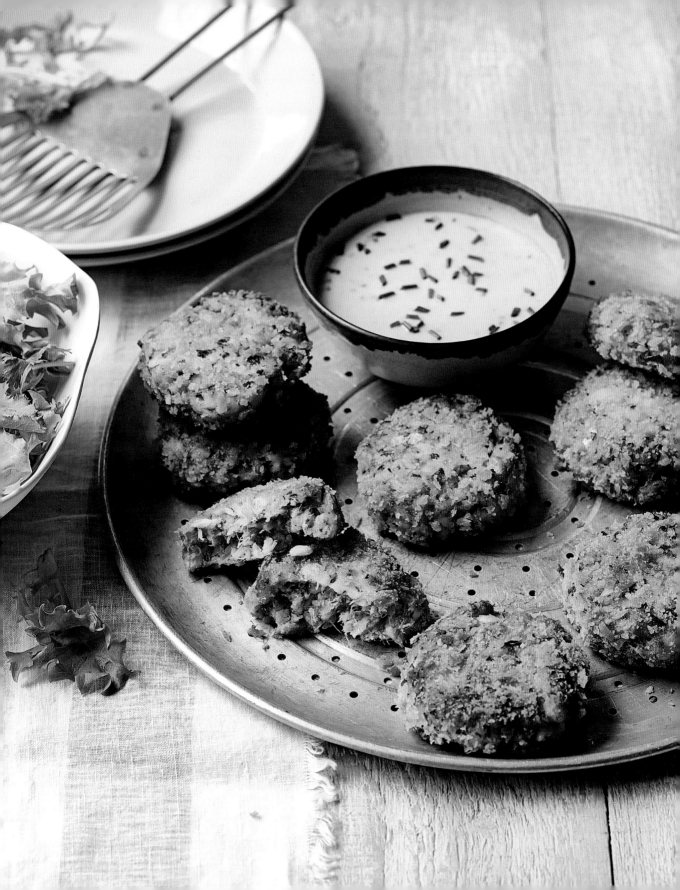

Cold Poached Salmon with Cucumber Quinoa Salad

1 unwaxed lemon, sliced

$\frac{1}{2}$ cup (120 ml) water

$\frac{1}{2}$ cup (120 ml) white wine

4 salmon fillets, about $4\frac{1}{2}$ oz (125 g) each

1 tablespoon capers

3 small cucumbers, diced

2 tablespoons finely sliced red onion, soaked in water for 10 minutes

$\frac{1}{2}$ yellow bell pepper, chopped

8 tablespoons (15 g) chopped dill

2 tablespoons chopped chives

2 cups (280 g) cooked quinoa

Himalayan salt and freshly ground black pepper, to taste

FOR THE DRESSING

4 tablespoons extra virgin olive oil

2 tablespoons champagne vinegar

Freshly squeezed juice of 1 clementine

Serves 4

This dish (pictured on the front cover of this book) is colorful, healthy, and so easy to entertain with. You can prepare everything the day before so it's simply a case of setting it out when you're ready to eat.

1 Put 4 slices of lemon, water, and white wine in a large skillet (frying pan). Place the salmon fillets on top of the lemon slices, skin side down. Bring the liquid to a simmer over a medium–high heat. Turn the heat to low, cover and cook for 5 minutes. Then turn off the heat, and let the fish continue to sit on the stove for a further 5 minutes while it continues to cook. This is a good way to prevent it from overcooking.

2 Transfer the salmon fillets to a plate, reserving the poaching liquid.

3 Add the capers, salt, and pepper to the poaching liquid and reduce by half over a medium heat to make a sauce. Drizzle the sauce over the salmon, cover, and chill in the refrigerator.

4 In a large mixing bowl, mix together the cucumber, red onion, bell pepper, 1 tablespoon each of the dill and chives, and the cooked quinoa. Make the dressing by whisking all of the ingredients together. Then drizzle over the quinoa salad and store in the refrigerator.

5 When you are ready to serve, plate the salmon with the quinoa salad and garnish with the reserved dill and chives.

Per serving: 512 kcals, 27.8 g fat (4.6 g saturates), 18.6 g carbohydrate (12.6 g sugars), 33.8 g protein, 4.2 g fiber, 0.5 g salt

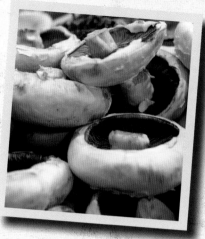

Mushroom Frittata

Who doesn't love breakfast for dinner? A frittata is typically started on the stove and finished in the oven, so use an ovenproof skillet (frying pan). You can use any kind of mushroom in this recipe, from white button to cremini (chestnut) to wild mushrooms.

2 tablespoons olive oil, divided

2 cups (125 g) sliced mushrooms

2 garlic cloves, minced

6 large (medium) eggs

2 large (medium) egg whites

2 tablespoons milk

Pinch of salt

½ cup (12 g) fresh basil leaves, torn

Serves 4–6

1 Preheat the oven to 450°F/230°C/Gas 8.

2 Heat 1 tablespoon of the oil in a 10–12-inch (25–30-cm) ovenproof skillet (frying pan) with a lid over medium–high heat. Add the mushrooms and garlic and sauté for 3–5 minutes until the mushrooms start to brown. Take off the heat.

3 Whisk together the eggs, egg whites, milk, and salt in a bowl.

4 Place the skillet back on the stove over medium heat and add the remaining oil. Pour in the egg mixture, add the basil, and swirl the skillet to distribute evenly. Turn the heat down to low and let the eggs cook for 2 minutes, then cover and let them cook for an additional 10 minutes.

5 Take the lid off, place the skillet in the preheated oven, and bake the frittata for 2–5 minutes until set.

Per serving (if serves 4): 183 kcals, 14.1 g fat (3.1 g saturates), 0.7 g carbohydrate (0.5 g sugars), 13.2 g protein, 0.3 g fiber, 0.6 g salt

Sweet Potato and Zucchini Pancakes

8 oz (225 g) orange-fleshed sweet potato, such as Garnet Yam, grated

1 small zucchini (courgette), finely grated

½ small onion, grated

2 eggs, beaten

½ teaspoon sea salt

¼ teaspoon freshly ground black pepper

⅛ teaspoon freshly grated nutmeg

½ cup (12 g) fresh basil leaves

1 tablespoon brown rice flour

1½ tablespoons extra virgin olive oil, for frying (you may need extra oil if frying the pancakes in batches)

TO SERVE

8 oz (225 g) smoked salmon

Greek yogurt

Chopped chives

Serves 4 (makes 16 small pancakes)

Those of us of the Jewish persuasion delight in potato pancakes (we call them latkes) on Hanukkah, the festival of lights; but they can be enjoyed at any time of year. Unlike the typical oil-drenched holiday fare, these pancakes need no blotting, as just a bit of olive oil is used for frying. If you like to change things up a bit, try serving the pancakes with applesauce instead of Greek yogurt.

1 Put the grated sweet potato, zucchini (courgette), and onion in a colander set over a bowl and press gently to squeeze out any excess moisture.

2 Whisk together the eggs, salt, pepper, and nutmeg in a large bowl. Add the sweet potato, zucchini (courgette), and onion, then add the basil and flour and stir with a rubber spatula until well mixed.

3 Heat the oil in a large skillet (frying pan) over medium heat. Drop heaped tablespoonfuls of the mixture into the skillet and flatten each portion with the back of the spoon—you may need to cook the pancakes in batches. Cook for 2 minutes on each side, or until golden brown on both sides. Transfer the pancakes to a platter, keeping them in a single layer.

4 Serve the pancakes hot or warm with smoked salmon, a dollop of Greek yogurt, and a sprinkling of chives.

Tip: Shred the basil just before adding it to retain its bright green color. Here's a convenient way to shred it: Stack the basil leaves, roll them into a cigar shape, and snip it with scissors or cut thin slices with a sharp knife.

Per serving: 320 kcals, 16.5 g fat (4.7 g saturates), 19.2 g carbohydrate (6 g sugars), 22.6 g protein, 2.2 g fiber, 2.6 g salt

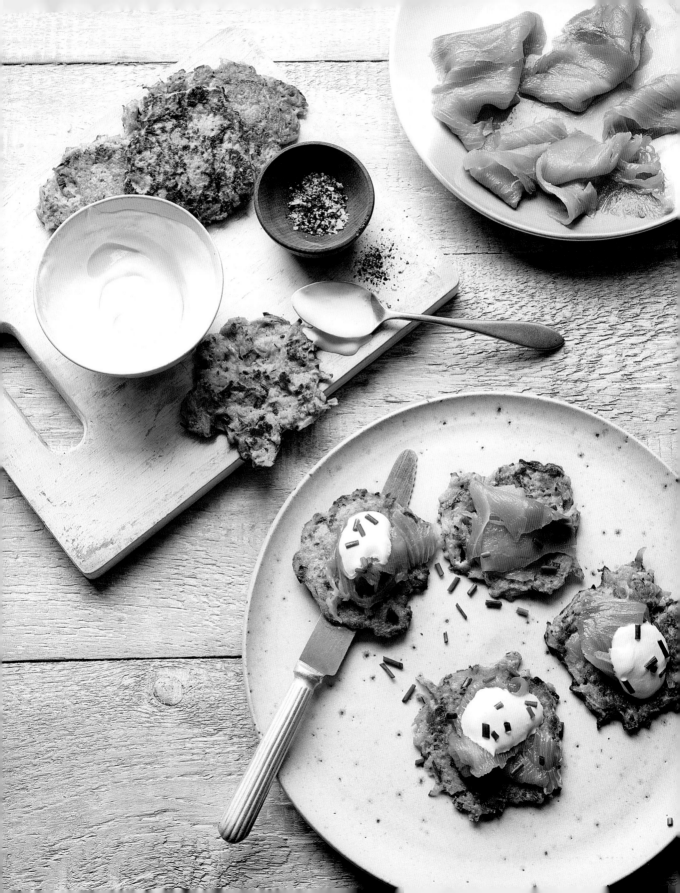

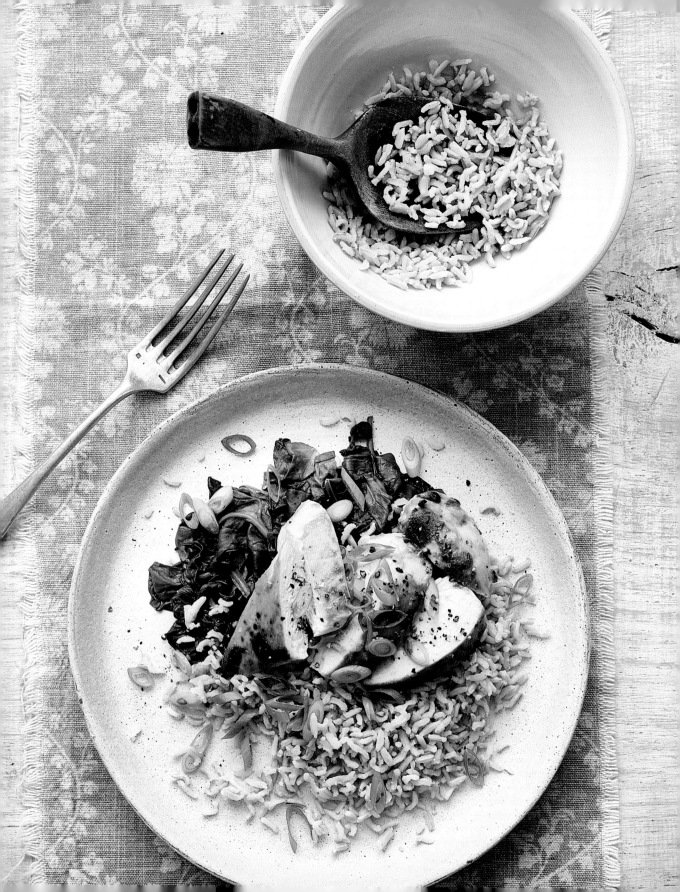

Broiled Miso-glazed Chicken Breast

2 tablespoons red miso (you can use a different type of miso if you prefer)

2 tablespoons mirin (or sake or dry sherry)

1 teaspoon ginger juice (see tip, below)

2 boneless and skinless chicken breasts, about 4–6 oz (120–175 g) each

TO SERVE

2 cups (270 g) cooked brown rice

1¹/₂ cups (340 g) cooked spinach

Sliced scallions (spring onions)

Serves 2

Rich red miso combined with sweet rice wine and zesty ginger turns a simple chicken dish into something that is robust and flavorful. If marinated in advance, a quick stint under the broiler (grill) makes this a must-have for your weeknight repertoire.

1 Mix together the miso, mirin, and ginger juice in a large bowl. Add the chicken breasts and turn them over until they are coated with the miso mixture. Cover with plastic wrap (clingfilm) and let stand in the refrigerator for at least 2 hours, or preferably overnight.

2 About 1 hour before you are ready to cook, remove the bowl of chicken from the refrigerator and let stand until it comes to room temperature.

3 Preheat the broiler (grill) to medium–high. Remove the chicken breasts from the miso mixture and place in a broiler-proof (grill-proof) pan. Broil (grill) the chicken for about 6 minutes on each side, or until cooked through. Be careful not to burn the chicken. Serve immediately with cooked brown rice and spinach, and sprinkled with scallions (spring onions).

Tip: To make ginger juice, grate a 2-inch (5-cm) piece of fresh ginger (there's no need to peel it), and squeeze the pulp into a small bowl.

Per serving: 500 kcals, 8.6 g fat (2 g saturates), 47 g carbohydrate (8 g sugars), 51 g protein, 8.2 g fiber, 2.6 g salt

Vegan Black-eyed Pea Chili

1 tablespoon extra virgin olive oil

1 teaspoon cumin seeds

2 cups (230 g) coarsely chopped onions

1 teaspoon dried oregano

$1/4$ teaspoon ground cinnamon

1 large green bell pepper, seeded and diced

$2^{1}/4$ cups dried black-eyed peas, picked over, rinsed, and drained

4 cups (950 ml) water

2–3 tablespoons chili powder

$1/4$ cup (65 g) mild or hot salsa (you may like to use more than this)

$1/4$ cup (10 g) finely chopped fresh cilantro (coriander) leaves

Salt

$1^{1}/2$ cups (225 g) cooked polenta, to serve

FOR THE GREEN SALAD

8 oz (225 g) romaine lettuce, torn into bite-sized pieces

1 tablespoon extra virgin olive oil

1 tablespoon balsamic vinegar

Freshly ground black pepper

Serves 6

Use a pressure cooker and fast-cooking black-eyed peas to make this tasty chili in no time at all. Alternatively, if you don't have a pressure cooker, you can cook the chili in a saucepan and increase the cooking time to 1 hour.

1 In an uncovered 6-quart (6-liter) stovetop pressure cooker, heat the oil over medium heat, then add the cumin seeds and let sizzle for about 5 seconds. Add the onions, oregano, cinnamon, bell pepper, black-eyed peas, water (stand back to avoid sputtering oil), and 2 tablespoons chili powder. Taste the liquid and add more chili powder if you like an intense chili flavor.

2 Cover and bring to high pressure over high heat. Reduce the heat until it is just hot enough to maintain high pressure and cook for 11 minutes. Turn off the heat and allow the pressure to come down naturally.

3 Remove the lid, tilting it away from you to allow any excess steam to escape. Stir in the salsa, tasting and adding a little more if you like, and season with salt. Simmer over low heat for a few minutes to allow the beans to pick up some of the salsa flavor. If the chili is too soupy, use an immersion blender to partially purée the mixture.

4 To make the salad, put the lettuce in a large bowl, drizzle over the oil and toss to coat, then sprinkle with the vinegar and toss again. Season to taste with salt and pepper.

5 When you are ready to serve, stir the cilantro (coriander) into the chili. Serve with the green salad and cooked polenta.

Per serving: 354 kcals, 5.9 g fat (1.1 g saturates), 52 g carbohydrate (7.3 g sugars), 21.2 g protein, 9.1 g fiber, 0.6 g salt

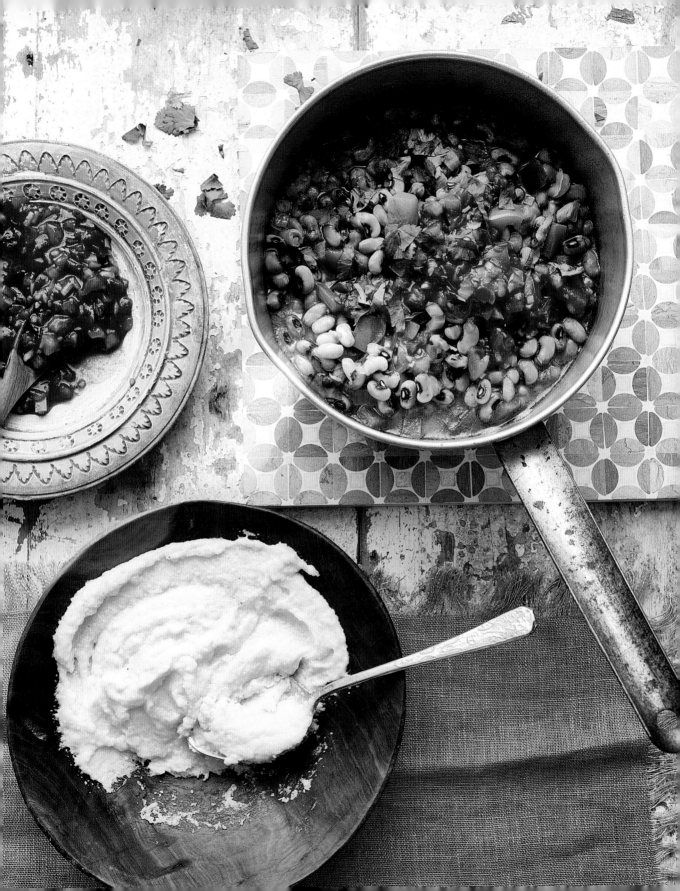

Bulked-up Miso Soup

4 cups (950 ml) water

2½ tablespoons white miso paste

½ x 1-lb (1 x 200-g) package firm tofu, chopped into bite-sized cubes

½ bunch kale (about ¾ lb/350 g), destemmed and leaves torn into bite-sized pieces

2 scallions (spring onions), white and green parts, thinly sliced

Serves 2–3

Miso soup is typically served as a starter to a meal. Here, it becomes a main course by being bulked up with larger chunks of tofu and kale. To make the soup even more substantial, stir in some cooked rice or soba noodles.

1 In a saucepan, bring the water to a boil. Reduce the heat to a gentle simmer.

2 Put the miso paste in a small bowl and pour a ladleful of the simmering water over the miso, whisking so it thins out and gets rid of most of the clumps.

3 Stir the miso paste mixture into the simmering water in the saucepan on the stove. Add the tofu, kale, and scallions (spring onions) and simmer for 10 minutes, or until the kale has softened.

Per serving (if serves 2): 278 kcals, 12.9 g fat (1.8 g saturates), 9.4 g carbohydrate (3.9 g sugars), 24.8 g protein, 8.6 g fiber, 2.3 g salt

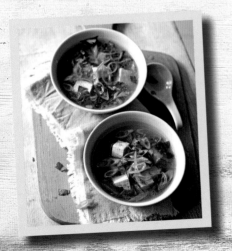

Turkey Chili

2 tablespoons olive oil

3 garlic cloves, minced

1 large yellow onion, diced

1 large red bell pepper, seeded and diced

¼ cup (50 g) diced celery

1 lb (450 g) ground (minced) lean turkey

4 tablespoons chili powder

½ teaspoon ground cumin

⅛ teaspoon ground cinnamon

⅛ teaspoon ground nutmeg

⅛ teaspoon cayenne pepper

½ teaspoon dried oregano

2 teaspoons freshly ground black pepper

1 x 28-oz can (2 x 400-g cans) diced tomatoes

1 cup (250 ml) low-sodium chicken stock

1 bay leaf

15 oz (400 g) cooked kidney or cannellini beans

Serves 4

Most chilis are made with high-fat ground (minced) beef. This recipe uses lean ground turkey as a healthier option, turning the chili into a delicious low-fat meal.

1 Heat the oil in a Dutch oven (casserole dish) over medium heat. Add the garlic, onion, bell pepper, and celery and cook for 3–5 minutes until the onions are translucent. Using a slotted spoon, transfer the vegetables to a plate and set aside.

2 Increase the heat to medium–high, add the turkey to the Dutch oven, and cook for 5–7 minutes until cooked through. Use a kitchen spoon to break the ground (minced) turkey into small pieces.

3 Return the vegetables to the Dutch oven and cook for 2 minutes. Add the spices, oregano, salt, and pepper and cook, stirring frequently, for a couple of minutes. Add the tomatoes, stock, bay leaf, and beans and simmer for 10 minutes. Remove and discard the bay leaf and serve.

Per serving: 298 kcals, 10.2 g fat (1.9 g saturates), 15.7 g carbohydrate (9.5 g sugars), 31.8 g protein, 6.8 g fiber, 1.6 g salt

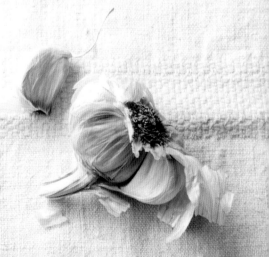

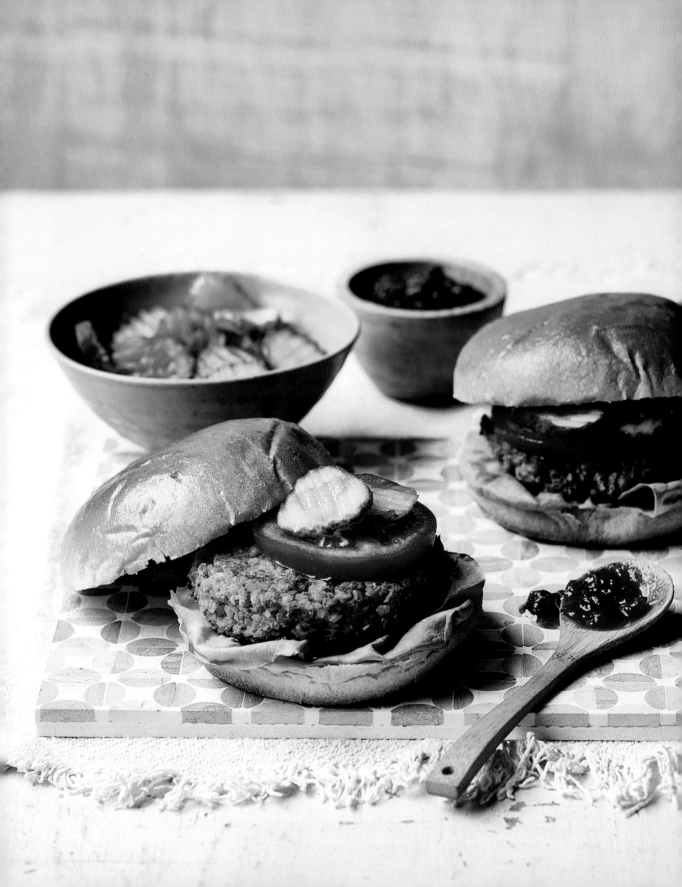

Veggie Burgers with Chickpeas and Tomato Chutney

1¼ cups (225 g) cooked bulgur wheat

1 x 15-oz (400-g) can chickpeas, rinsed and drained

¼ cup (25 g) grated Cheddar cheese (use non-dairy cheese if you prefer)

2 tablespoons tomato chutney or ketchup

Nonstick cooking spray, for greasing

TO SERVE

5 burger buns, split in half

Your favorite toppings, such as sliced tomato, sliced gherkin, and lettuce

Serves 5

Feel free to substitute brown rice or couscous instead of the bulgur wheat. You may also use mashed black beans or white beans in place of the chickpeas. For a lighter meal, serve the burgers on iceburg lettuce leaves or large tomato slices instead of buns.

1 Preheat the oven to 350°F/180°C/Gas 4. Grease a baking pan with nonstick cooking spray.

2 Put the bulgur wheat, chickpeas, Cheddar cheese, and tomato chutney or ketchup in a bowl and mash together until they're well blended. Using your hands, shape the mixture into 5 patties—make sure they are all uniform in size to ensure they cook evenly.

3 Place the patties in the prepared baking pan and bake in the preheated oven for 25 minutes, then turn them over and return to the oven for an additional 15 minutes. Serve the patties in burger buns and add your favorite toppings.

Per serving: 315 kcals, 7.2 g fat (2.1 g saturates), 47 g carbohydrate (4.5 g sugars), 12.6 g protein, 5.2 g fiber, 1.1 g salt

Fish Tacos with Herby Slaw

1 tablespoon olive oil

1 lb (450 g) skinless mild-flavored fish fillets, such as cod

1/2 teaspoon chili powder

FOR THE HERBY SLAW

1/2 head cabbage, shredded

1 cup (20 g) fresh cilantro (coriander) leaves, chopped

Juice of 1 lime

TO SERVE

8 x 6-inch (15-cm) corn tortillas, warmed

1 large tomato, chopped

Serves 4

Skip the line at the local taco joint and make your own tacos at home. The shredded cabbage gives the slaw its low-carb crunch, while the cilantro (coriander) and lime juice add freshness. To make these tacos even more special, serve with avocado slices or guacamole.

1 Heat the oil in a large skillet (frying pan) over medium–high heat. Add the fish, sprinkle with the chili powder, and cook for 2–3 minutes on each side until the fish starts to whiten around the outside and is easily flaked with a fork. Take off the heat and let cool slightly, then gently tear or slice the fish into strips or bite-sized pieces.

2 In a large bowl, stir together the cabbage, cilantro (coriander), and the lime juice.

3 To serve, divide the fish among 8 warmed corn tortillas, add a large spoonful of herby slaw to each taco, and top with the chopped tomato.

Per serving: 397 kcals, 9.6 g fat (2 g saturates), 45 g carbohydrate (10.8 g sugars), 28.6 g protein, 10.9 g fiber, 1 g salt

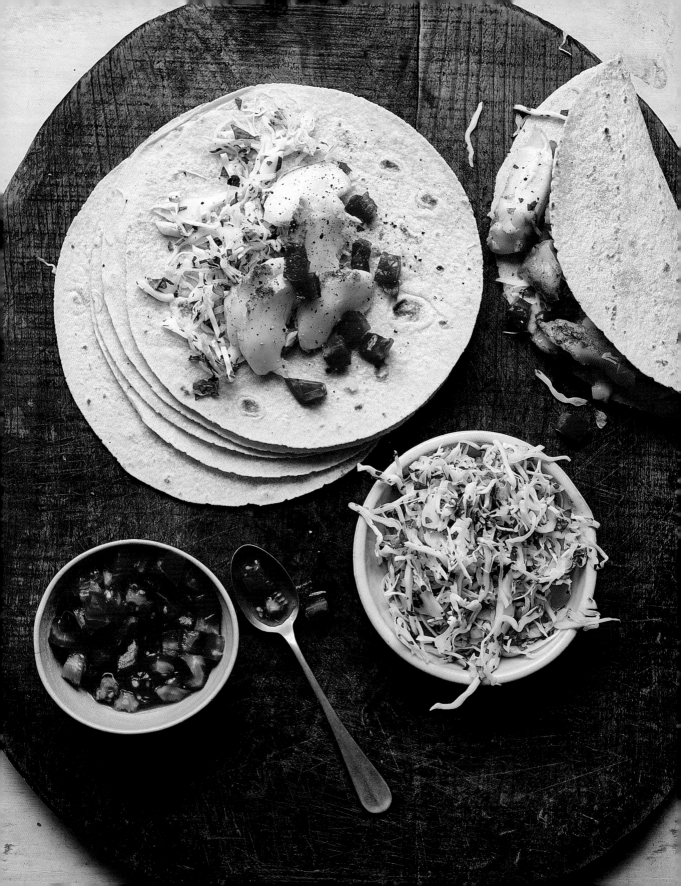

Chicken, Apple, and Arugula Patties

2 lb (900 g) ground (minced) dark-meat chicken

1 cup (50 g) arugula (rocket) or spinach, finely chopped

1 cup (100 g) peeled and diced apple

²/₃ cup (100 g) finely chopped onion

1 teaspoon crushed fennel seeds

¹/₂ teaspoon ground cumin

¹/₂ teaspoon salt

¹/₂ teaspoon freshly ground pepper

A few drops of freshly squeezed lemon juice

Extra virgin olive oil, for brushing

8 burger buns, split in half

Serves 8

These chicken patties are ideal for a protein rush. Apple, which is commonly added to sausages, adds a pleasant, sweet taste to the patties that isn't overpowering. The patties are quick and easy to make and store well in the freezer.

1 Mix the chicken, arugula (rocket) or spinach, apple, onion, fennel seeds, cumin, salt, pepper, and lemon juice together in a large bowl. Using your hands, shape the mixture into 8 patties—make sure they are all uniform in size to ensure they cook evenly.

2 Heat a dry grill (griddle) pan over medium heat and then brush it with oil. Add the patties and cook for about 4 minutes on each side, until browned on both sides and cooked through—the meat should feel firm when you press on it with your finger. (You may need to reduce the heat to medium–low and cook for a little longer if the patties are browned on the outside but the meat is not cooked through.) Serve the patties in burger buns.

Per serving: 339 kcals, 11.8 g fat (3.1 g saturates), 29.3 g carbohydrate (3.5 g sugars), 28 g protein, 1.5 g fiber, 1.4 g salt

Chicken and Peppers with Linguini

This recipe provides a healthy twist on the traditional Italian sausage with peppers dish. Chicken breasts are used instead of sausages, and whole wheat pasta replaces the hot dog bun or roll, making this dish low in fat but high in flavor.

1 Heat a large sauté pan over medium heat. Once the pan is hot, add the oil and chicken and sauté for 5 minutes. Using a slotted spoon, transfer the chicken to a plate and set aside.

2 Add the onions, garlic, and bell peppers to the pan and cook, stirring occasionally, for 2 minutes. Add the tomato paste (purée) and cook for 1 minute, stirring frequently to avoid burning the tomato paste, then add the tomatoes, salt, and basil. Return the chicken to the pan and cook for 15 minutes or until cooked through. Serve with cooked whole wheat linguine.

Per serving: 258 kcals, 4.8 g fat (1.3 g saturates), 14.2 g carbohydrate (7.5 g sugars), 38.1 g protein, 2.8 g fiber, 1.9 g salt

1 tablespoon olive oil

4 boneless and skinless chicken breasts, about 4–6 oz (120–175 g) each, sliced

1 cup (130 g) sliced onions

1 tablespoon minced garlic

1 cup (75 g) sliced green bell peppers

1¹/₂ tablespoons tomato paste (purée)

8 oz (225 g) canned diced tomatoes

1 teaspoon salt

1 tablespoon fresh chopped basil

1¹/₃ cups (85 g) cooked whole wheat linguine

Serves 4

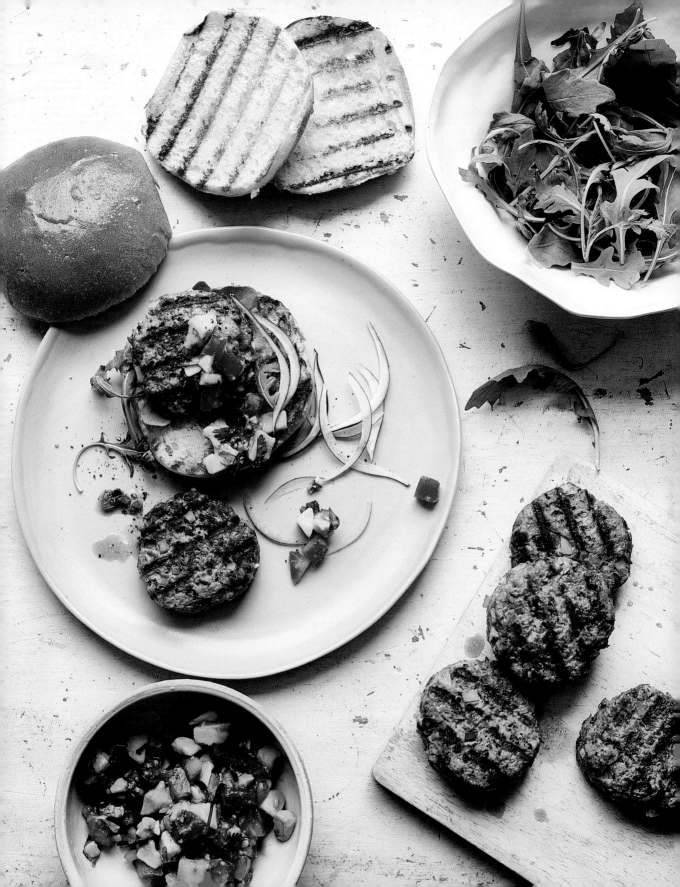

Shrimp Stir Fry

1½ tablespoons vegetable or peanut oil, divided

1 lb (450 g) raw shrimp (prawns), shelled, peeled, and deveined

1½ tablespoons minced garlic

1 tablespoon minced fresh ginger

3 cups (180 g) broccoli florets

1½ cups (175 g) sliced carrots

2 cups (160 g) snow peas (mangetout), stems and strings removed

1 tablespoon oyster or hoisin sauce

1⅓ cups (180 g) cooked brown rice

Serves 4

Stir frys are typically high in fat as the meat or protein is shallow-fried in oil and then cooked with vegetables, with additional oil added throughout the cooking process. The following recipe uses a lean protein— the shrimp (prawns)—and very little oil.

1 Heat a large sauté pan over medium–high heat. Once the pan is hot, add 1 tablespoon of the oil and the shrimp (prawns) and cook, stirring frequently, until the shrimp start to turn pink. Using a slotted spoon, transfer the shrimp to a plate and set aside.

2 Add the remaining oil to the pan, then add the garlic and ginger and stir-fry for about 15 seconds. Add broccoli, carrots, and snow peas (mangetout) and stir-fry for 2–4 minutes until the vegetables begin to soften but still retain some bite.

3 Add the oyster or hoisin sauce, stirring constantly, then return the shrimp to the pan and stir-fry for an additional 1 minute, or until the shrimp and vegetables are evenly coated with the sauce. Serve immediately with cooked brown rice.

Per serving: 224 kcals, 3.4 g fat (0.5 g saturates), 20.2 g carbohydrate (6.5 g sugars), 25.7 g protein, 5.3 g fiber, 1.6 g salt

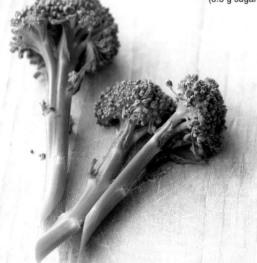

Chicken and Vegetable Soup

Soups are an easy way to combine protein and vegetables in one dish. This recipe uses extra-lean meat and vegetables to create a high-protein, high-fiber, and low-fat dish.

4 boneless and skinless chicken breasts, about 4–6 oz (120–175 g) each, cut into 1-inch (2.5-cm) cubes

1½ tablespoons olive oil, divided

1 small onion, cut into ½-inch (1-cm) cubes

1 carrot, cut into ½-inch (1-cm) cubes

1 celery stalk, cut into ½-inch (1-cm) cubes

4 bay leaves

1½ tablespoons dried thyme

1 tablespoon dried parsley

2½ quarts (2.35 liters) low- or no-sodium chicken stock

4 cups (600 g) frozen mixed vegetables

Salt and freshly ground black pepper

Serves 4

1 Put the chicken in a bowl and season with 1 teaspoon each of salt and pepper.

2 Heat 1 tablespoon of the oil in a Dutch oven (casserole dish) over medium heat. Add the chicken and sauté for 5 minutes, stirring occasionally. Remove the chicken from the Dutch oven and set aside.

3 Add the remaining oil and the onion, carrot, and celery to the Dutch oven and sauté for 3 minutes, then add the herbs and cook for 2–3 minutes until the onions are translucent.

4 Pour over the stock, then return the chicken to the Dutch oven, cover, and simmer over medium heat for 30 minutes. Add the frozen mixed vegetables and simmer, uncovered, for an additional 15–20 minutes until the vegetables are tender and the chicken is cooked through. Taste and adjust the seasoning if necessary. Serve hot.

Per serving: 353 kcals, 10.2 g fat (2 g saturates), 21.1 g carbohydrate (14.5 g sugars), 41 g protein, 7.8 g fiber, 1.1 g salt

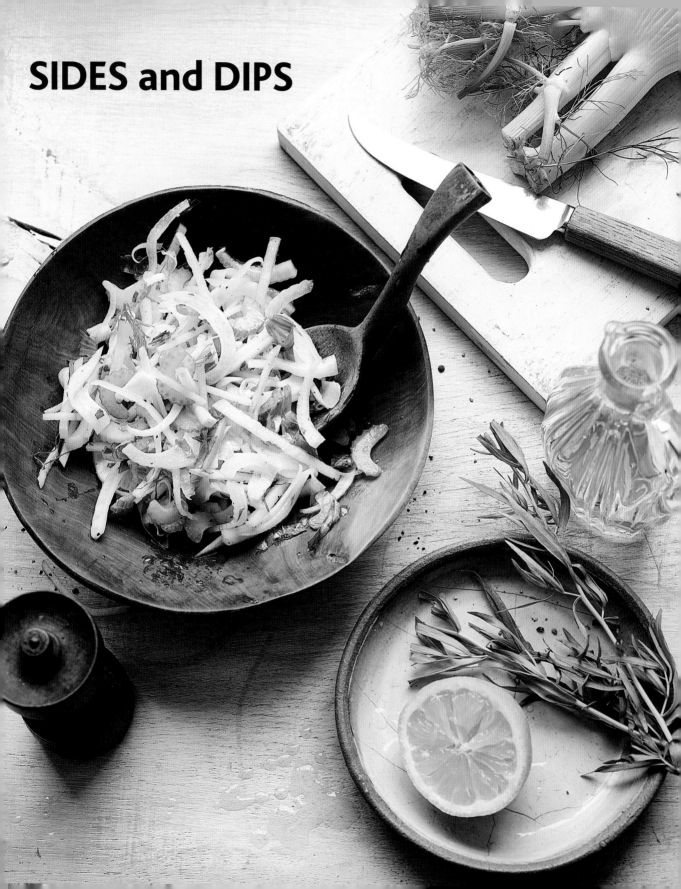

SIDES and DIPS

Apple, Celery, and Fennel Slaw

This slaw is one of the freshest and cleanest I know. I eat it year round, not just in the warmer months. When served with stews and richer meat dishes, it is a welcome crisp accompaniment.

1 Mix together the oil, vinegar, tarragon, lemon juice, and sugar in a bowl. Add the celery and celery leaves, fennel and fennel fronds, and apple and toss to coat. Season with salt and pepper.

Per serving: 122 kcals, 9.9 g fat (1.4 g saturates), 5.9 g carbohydrate (5.8 g sugars), 0.8 g protein, 2.5 g fiber, 0.2 g salt

3 tablespoons extra virgin olive oil

3 tablespoons apple cider vinegar

2 tablespoons chopped fresh tarragon

2 teaspoons lemon juice

1/4 teaspoon natural sugar, such as coconut sugar

3 celery stalks, thinly sliced, plus 1/4 cup (12 g) celery leaves

2 small fennel bulbs, thinly sliced crosswise, plus 1 tablespoon chopped fennel fronds

1 apple (choose a crisp and firm apple variety, like Pink Lady, Gala, or Granny Smith), cut into long, thin strips

Salt and freshly ground black pepper

Serves 4

Low-fat Coleslaw

1 cup (135 g) grated carrots

6 cups (350 g) grated red cabbage

1 small shallot, sliced

1/4 cup (60 ml) white balsamic vinegar

Salt and freshly ground black pepper

1/2 teaspoon celery seeds

Serves 4

Typically, coleslaw is made with mayonnaise; however, this low-fat version uses white balsamic vinegar as a base.

1 Mix all the ingredients together in a large bowl. Cover with plastic wrap (clingfilm) and refrigerate for at least 15 minutes before serving.

Per serving: 57 kcals, 0.4 g fat (0.1 g saturates), 8.7 g carbohydrate (8.2 g sugars), 2 g protein, 4.7 g fiber, 0.2 g salt

Roasted Cumin Carrots

Roasting vegetables makes them irresistible, and mixing ground cumin into the olive oil adds a ton of flavor to these roasted carrots.

3 tablespoons olive oil

2 teaspoons ground cumin

Pinch of salt

Pinch of freshly ground black pepper

1 bunch carrots (about 1–1½ lb/ 450–675 g), trimmed of their greens and cut into finger-sized sticks

Serves 4

1 Preheat the oven to 425°F/220°C/Gas 7. Line a baking sheet with parchment (baking) paper.

2 In a small bowl, mix together the oil, cumin, salt, and pepper

3 Spread out the carrots on the prepared baking sheet. Pour the cumin oil over the carrots and then, using your hands, turn over the carrots until they are evenly coated with the cumin oil. Bake in the preheated oven for 25–30 minutes, stirring or turning the carrots halfway through the cooking time, until the carrots start browning and are just tender.

Per serving: 156 kcals, 10.3 g fat (1.5 g saturates), 11.5 g carbohydrate (10.5 g sugars), 0.9 g protein, 6 g fiber, 0.2 g salt

Broccoli Rabe with Chipped Garlic

1 tablespoon olive oil

2 garlic cloves, thinly sliced

⅛ teaspoon red chili flakes

1 x 11-oz (315-g) bunch of broccoli rabe, roughly chopped into bite-sized pieces

Salt and freshly ground black pepper

Serves 2–4

Broccoli rabe is a leafy vegetable that some people may think of as bitter tasting. Sautéing it with thinly sliced "garlic chips" cuts through some of that bitterness. If you can't source broccoli rabe, substitute Swiss chard or a similar leafy green.

1 Heat the oil in a large skillet (frying pan) with a lid over medium–high heat. Add the garlic and chili and sauté for 30 seconds–1 minute, then add the broccoli rabe and sauté for 2 minutes.

2 Turn the heat down to medium–low, carefully add 2–4 tablespoons water to the skillet, cover, and steam the broccoli rabe for 2–4 minutes until the leaves are bright green and wilted and the stems are tender. Season with salt and pepper.

Per serving (if serves 2): 102 kcals, 6.9 g fat (0.9 g saturates), 4.7 g carbohydrate (4.6 g sugars), 3.1 g protein, 3.8 g fiber, 1 g salt

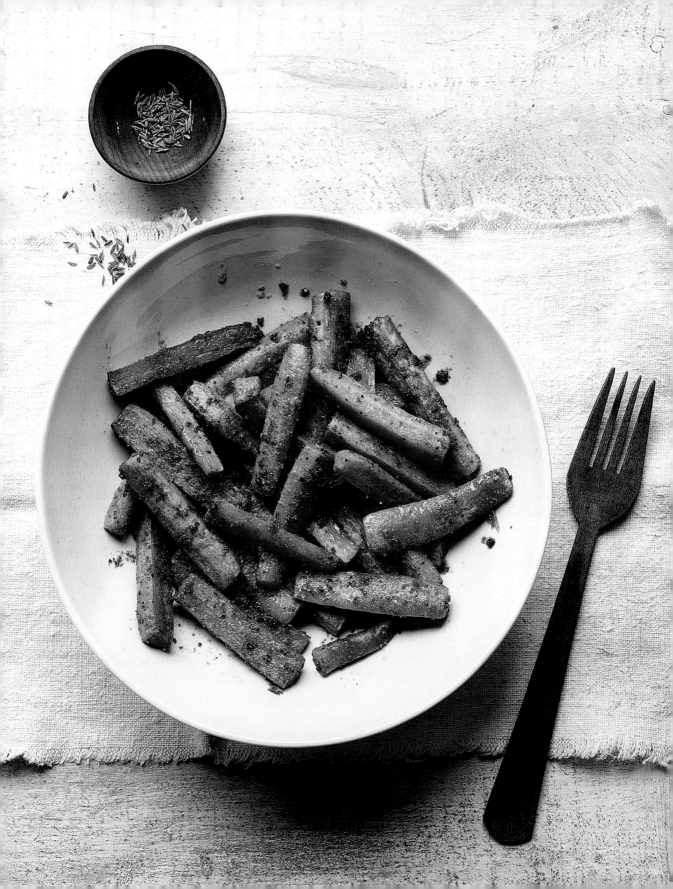

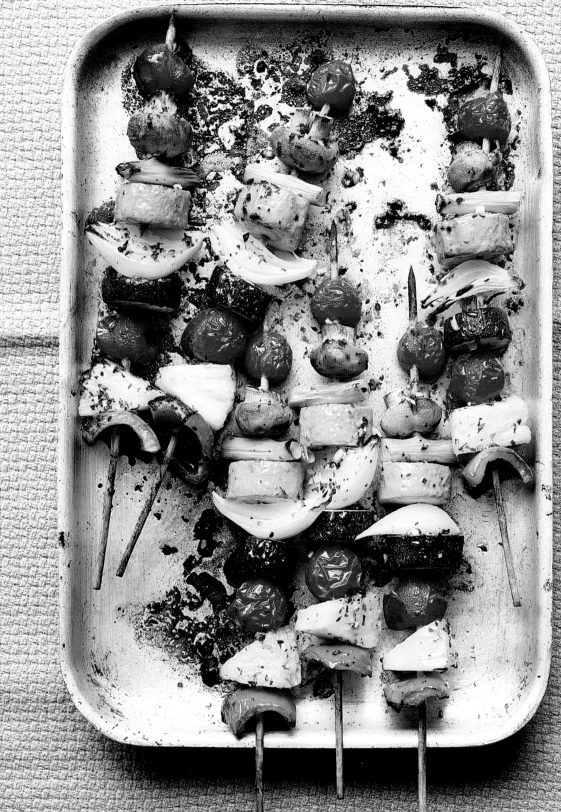

Roasted Vegetable and Pineapple Skewers

These skewers are fun to prepare, great as appetizers at a party, and a different way to get kids to eat their vegetables. This recipe is can be adapted to include your favorite vegetables.

1 Preheat the oven to 425°F/220°C/Gas 7.

2 Whisk together the oil, lemon juice, garlic, oregano, and basil in a small bowl. Set aside.

3 To assemble, thread and divide the onions, scallions (spring onions), bell pepper, zucchini (courgettes), mushrooms, tomatoes, and pineapple between 8 skewers, alternating softer and harder vegetables.

4 Place the vegetable skewers on a baking sheet and brush them with half the herby oil. Roast in the preheated oven for 10–15 minutes, or until the vegetables are soft, turning the skewers halfway through the cooking time and brushing them with the remaining herby oil.

Per serving: 91 kcals, 6.7 g fat (1 g saturates), 4.6 g carbohydrate (4.1 g sugars), 1.6 g protein, 2.3 g fiber, trace salt

$^{1}/_{4}$ cup (60 ml) olive oil

Juice of 1 small lemon

2 small garlic cloves, minced

$^{1}/_{2}$ teaspoon dried oregano

$^{1}/_{2}$ teaspoon dried basil

1 cup (115 g) pearl onions (whole) or yellow onions (chopped)

3–4 scallions (spring onions), cut into $^{3}/_{4}$–1 inch (2–2.5-cm) slices

1 green bell pepper, seeded and cut into 1-inch (2.5-cm) slices

1 green zucchini (courgette), cut into $^{1}/_{2}$-inch (1-cm) slices

1 yellow zucchini (courgette), cut into $^{1}/_{2}$-inch (1-cm) slices

1 cup (70 g) button mushrooms

1 cup (170 g) cherry tomatoes

$^{1}/_{2}$ cup (80 g) fresh pineapple, cut into 1-inch (2.5-cm) chunks

Serves 8

Yellow Cauliflower "Rice"

1 head cauliflower, broken into florets and any tough stems cut off and discarded

1 teaspoon olive oil

1 teaspoon ground turmeric

Serves 6

Traditional yellow rice is yellow in color because it contains chicken stock. This non-starchy vegetable "rice" is made from grated cauliflower, and it gets its vibrant color from the turmeric, a spice that is being studied for its possible anti-inflammatory properties.

1 Put the cauliflower in a food processor and pulse until the pieces have become the size of rice grains. Alternatively, carefully grate the florets with a cheese grater.

2 Heat the oil in a large nonstick skillet (frying pan) over medium–high heat. When the oil is hot, add the turmeric, followed by the cauliflower "rice." Sauté for about 3–4 minutes, stirring frequently, just until the "rice" has warmed through.

Per serving: 59 kcals, 1.3 g fat (0.2 g saturates), 6.4 g carbohydrate (4.3 g sugars), 3.8 g protein, 2.7 g fiber, trace salt

Parmesan Asparagus

2¼ lbs (1 kg) asparagus

2–3 tablespoons olive oil

¼ cup (20 g) grated Parmesan cheese

Serves 4

This dish would be a delicious accompaniment to steak, chicken, or fish, or you could serve it with slices of Serrano ham for a lighter meal.

1 Preheat the oven to 350°F/180°C/Gas 4.

2 Break off the tough part at the base of the asparagus spears and discard. Place the asparagus in a casserole dish and pour over the oil.

3 Bake in the preheated oven for 15 minutes. Turn over the asparagus and sprinkle the Parmesan over the top. Return to the oven and bake for an additional 10 minutes.

Per serving: 179 kcals, 12.5 g fat (2.6 g saturates), 5 g carbohydrate (4.8 g sugars), 9.1 g protein, 4.3 g fiber, 0.1 g salt

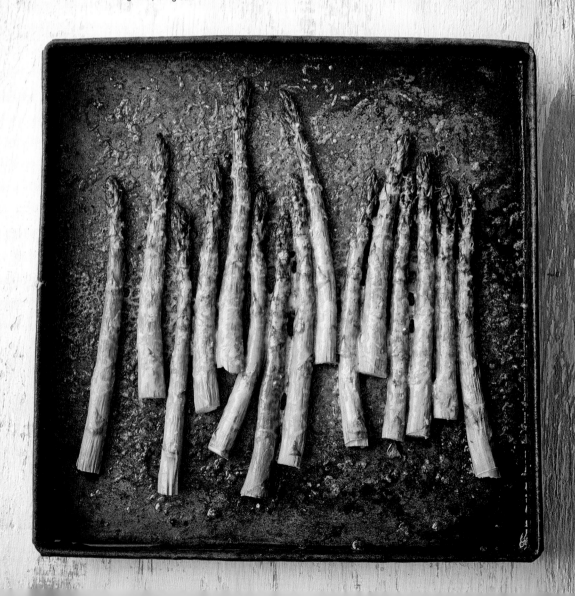

Hummus

1 small garlic clove, minced

2 tablespoons minced onion

1 tablespoon lemon juice

1½ cups (200 g) canned chickpeas, rinsed and drained

¼ cup (60 g) tahini

2 tablespoons olive oil

½ teaspoon ground cumin

1 teaspoon salt

½ teaspoon white pepper (you can use black pepper if white pepper is not available)

2–3 tablespoons water

A selection of prepared fresh vegetables, such as carrot sticks, celery sticks, cherry tomatoes, and broccoli florets, to serve

Serves 6

Hummus is a Mediterranean dish that can be served as a dip for vegetables or used as a sandwich spread. Made with chickpeas, which are high in protein and fiber, hummus is a healthier alternative to cream-based dips such as ranch or blue cheese.

1 Mix together the garlic, onion, and lemon juice in a small bowl. Set aside.

2 Put the remaining ingredients in a food processor or blender and blend until smooth. Add the garlic mixture and blend until smooth. Serve the hummus with a selection of prepared fresh vegetables.

Per serving of hummus without the vegetables: 136 kcals, 11.1 g fat (1.6 g saturates), 5.6 g carbohydrate (0.5 g sugars), 4.4 g protein, 2.6 g fiber, 0.9 g salt

Simple Mayonnaise

Once you've mastered the basic mayonnaise recipe, it's easy to whip up variations. Try adding a little chili sauce, a few drops of truffle oil, or some chopped fresh herbs.

1 Put the egg in a blender cup or large beaker and then pour the oil over it. Let sit for a minute or two, then add the mustard, lemon juice, salt, and pepper.

2 Put an immersion blender into the cup or beaker so that it sits at the bottom and then start the blender. Within a few seconds you should be able to see mayonnaise forming at the bottom of the bowl. Continue to blend, moving the immersion blender around to mix in the remaining oil, until you have a smooth, glossy mayonnaise.

3 If you're not using the mayonnaise straight away, cover and store in the refrigerator. It will keep for 5 days.

1 egg

1 cup plus 1 tablespoon (250 ml) mild olive, cold-pressed coconut, avocado, walnut, or sunflower seed oil

1 teaspoon Dijon mustard

A few drops of freshly squeezed lemon juice

Pinch of salt

Pinch of freshly ground black pepper

Makes 1¼ cups (225 g)

Tip: Each type of oil has a slightly different taste, so use whichever one you prefer. My favorite option is a mixture of half mild olive oil and half cold-pressed coconut oil, which has the most neutral flavor.

Per level tablespoon: 100 kcals, 10.9 g fat (1.6 g saturates), trace carbohydrate (trace sugars), 0.4 g protein, 0 g fiber, 0.1 g salt

Radish-spiked Yogurt Dip

1 cup (215 g) plain yogurt

1/3 cup chopped fresh herbs, such as mint, flat-leaf parsley, or cilantro (coriander)

2 tablespoons finely chopped red onion

1 tablespoon lemon juice

1 cup (50 g) coarsely grated red radishes

Salt, for sprinkling

Olive oil, for drizzling

Makes 1¹/₂ cups (350 g)

This yogurt dip (pictured top left) uses grated radishes instead of the more traditional grated cucumber. Use Greek-style yogurt if you would like additional protein. Serve with freshly sliced vegetables, including extra sliced radishes, or with whole wheat pita bread or crackers.

1 Put the yogurt, herbs, onion, lemon juice, and radishes in a bowl and mix well. Add a sprinkling of salt and a drizzle of oil.

For the whole batch: 229 kcals, 10.8 g fat (4.8 g saturates), 20.2 g carbohydrate (19 g sugars), 12.9 g protein, 0.7 g fiber, 1.5 g salt

Smoky Edamame Dip with Cucumber "Chips"

This high-protein creamy, salty, nutty, and smoky dip (pictured bottom right) is versatile enough that you can adjust the cumin and coriander and shoyu or tamari (soy sauce) to your desired balance of the three tastes. If you like a dip with a kick, add some chili powder to the mix. It could also be used as a sandwich spread.

1 lb (450 g) frozen shelled edamame

2 tablespoons shoyu or tamari (soy sauce)

1 tablespoon sesame oil

1 teaspoon ground cumin

1¹/₂ teaspoons ground coriander

¹/₄ teaspoon ground cinnamon

¹/₄ teaspoon salt

3 cucumbers (I like to use English cucumbers but you can use any variety you prefer)

Serves 4

1 Bring a large pan of water to a boil and cook the edamame according to the package directions. Drain, reserving ¼–½ cup (60–120 ml) of the cooking water.

2 Combine the shoyu or tamari (soy sauce), oil, spices, and salt in a food processor or blender and blend until smooth, adding a little of the reserved cooking water to obtain the desired creamy consistency. Transfer the dip to a small serving bowl.

3 Cut the cucumbers into slices about ⅛–¼ inch/3–5 mm thick. Arrange the cucumbers on a serving platter and serve with the dip. Guests can use the cucumber slices to scoop out the dip in lieu of chips.

Per serving: 227 kcals, 11.1 g fat (0.4 g saturates), 9.9 g carbohydrate (8.1 g sugars), 16.8 g protein, 8.6 g fiber, 1.7 g salt

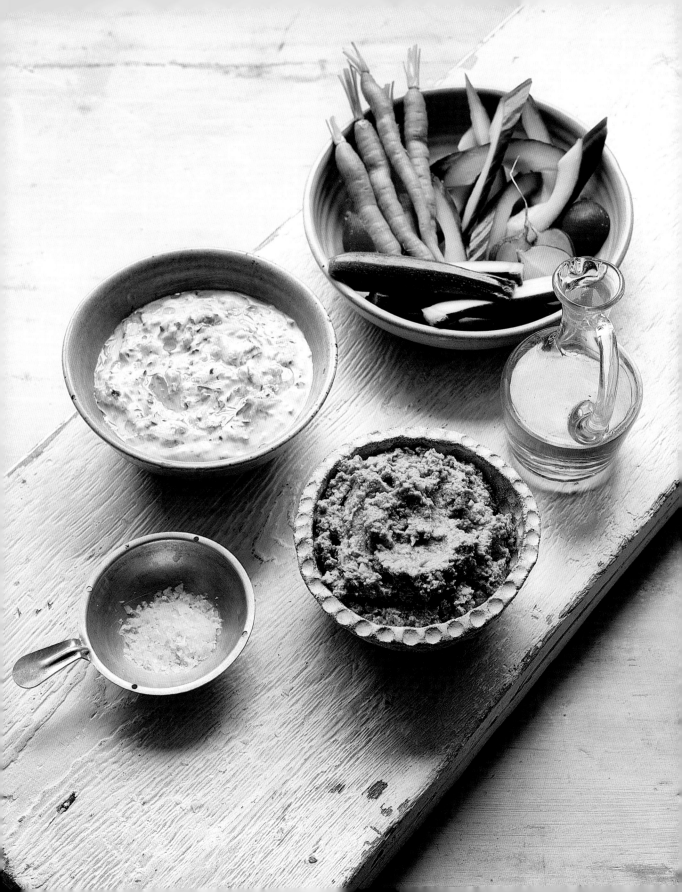

DESSERTS and TREATS

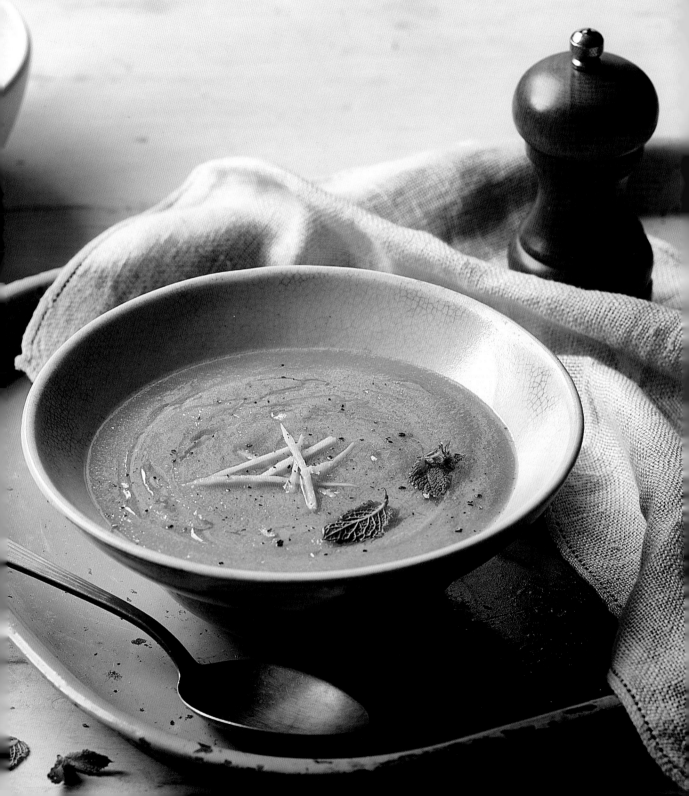

Cold Melon Soup with Ginger

This soup is amazingly refreshing. Not only is it low in calories but it also has the additional benefit of containing ginger, which boosts the immune system.

2 cantaloupe melons, peeled, seeded, and cut into chunks

1 tablespoon extra virgin olive oil

1 teaspoon grated fresh ginger

Pinch of fleur de sel

1-inch (2.5-cm) piece of fresh ginger, peeled and cut into strips, to garnish

Fresh mint leaves, to garnish

Serves 4

1 Put the melons, oil, ginger, and fleur de sel in a food processor or blender and blend until smooth.

2 Pour the soup into bowls and garnish with strips of fresh ginger and mint leaves.

Per serving: 86 kcals, 3.5 g fat (0.5 g saturates), 11.3 g carbohydrate (10.9 g sugars), 1.1 g protein, 2.7 g fiber, 0.2 g salt

Apples, Walnuts, and Peanut Butter

2 apples (choose a firm apple variety, such as Granny Smith)

2 tablespoons smooth peanut butter

1 cup (135 g) walnut pieces

Serves 4

This high-energy, low-sugar combination is a great healthy dessert or snack for diabetics (and everyone!).

1 Peel, core, and slice the apples.

2 Divide the apple slices among plates and then add a small dollop of peanut butter and a heap of walnuts to each plate. Let your guests dip the apple slices in the peanut butter and then the walnuts.

Per serving: 325 kcals, 27.3 g fat (3.6 g saturates), 10.8 g carbohydrate (10 g sugars), 7.1 g protein, 3.4 g fiber, 0.1 g salt

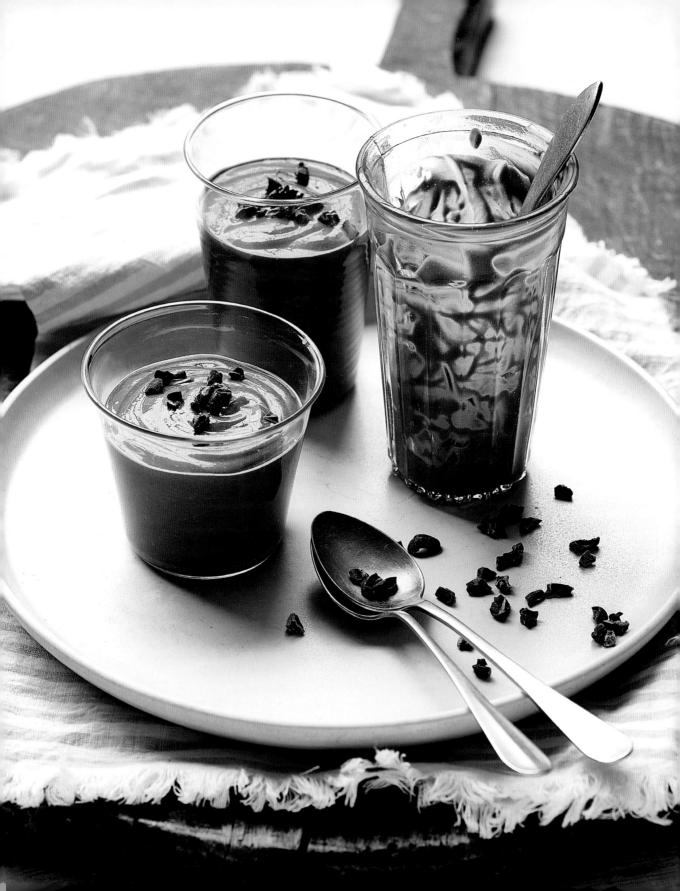

PB&T Chocolate Pudding

Silken tofu gives this pudding body, and it adds protein too. Don't worry, the addition of the cocoa powder and peanut butter means that no one will know you snuck in the tofu.

1 lb (450 g) silken tofu

1/3 cup (30 g) unsweetened cocoa powder

1/4 cup (60 ml) maple syrup or agave nectar

1 tablespoon vanilla extract

3 tablespoons peanut butter

Serves 4–6

1 Combine all the ingredients in a food processor or blender and blend until smooth.

2 Pour the pudding mixture into mini cups or bowls and enjoy.

Per serving (if serves 6): 216 kcals, 12.5 g fat (3.3 g saturates), 15.9 g carbohydrate (11.2 g sugars), 10.2 g protein, 2 g fiber, 0.2 g salt

Banana Oat Bars

3 bananas

1 teaspoon vanilla extract

2 cups (190 g) rolled or quick oats

1/2 cup (125 g) chopped nuts or seeds, such as walnuts, almonds, pecans, sunflower seeds, or pumpkin seeds

1/4 cup (40 g) chopped dried fruit, such as cherries, apricots, dates, figs, or raisins

Makes 6 bars

Many store-bought and even homemade granola bars contain a lot of added sugar. These bars get most of their sugar from the mashed bananas, which also act as a glue to help the bars to stick together.

1 Preheat the oven to 350°F/180°C/Gas 4. Line a 9 x 9-inch (23 x 23-cm) baking pan with parchment (baking) paper.

2 Peel the bananas and place them in a bowl. Mash them very well. Add the vanilla and then stir in the oats, nuts or seeds, and dried fruit. Tip the mixture into the prepared baking pan and use the back of a spoon to press it down lightly so the surface is even.

3 Bake in the preheated oven for 30 minutes, or just until the edges start to brown. Let cool in the baking pan, then cut into 6 bars. The banana oat bars will keep for 4–5 days in an airtight container or can be frozen for up to 3 months.

Per serving: 312 kcals, 12.9 g fat (2 g saturates), 37.2 g carbohydrate (14.7 g sugars), 9.1 g protein, 4.6 g fiber, trace salt

Lemon and Coconut Bliss Balls

⅔ cup (50 g) desiccated unsweetened coconut, plus extra for coating

Scant ½ cup (70 g) almond flour

3½ tablespoons (50 ml) coconut oil

½ teaspoon pure vanilla powder

Grated zest and juice of ½ unwaxed lemon

Makes about 10 balls

These no-bake treats are perfect as a snack, and can even be served as dessert. The sweet coconut and tangy lemon flavors will send your senses off to a far-away Caribbean island!

1 Put all the ingredients in a bowl and mix together. Using your hands, roll small portions of the mixture into bite-sized balls.

2 Spread out some extra coconut in a shallow dish and roll the balls in the coconut to coat.

3 Place the balls on a plate or tray and chill in the refrigerator for an hour or so. The balls can be stored in an airtight container for up to 7 days in the refrigerator.

Per ball: 121 kcals, 11.7 g fat (7.1 g saturates), 0.9 g carbohydrate (0.7 g sugars), 1.8 g protein, 2.1 g fiber, trace salt

Coconut Macaroons

Often the simplest recipes are the most delicious. Such is the case with these coconut macaroons, the perfect occasional treat.

1 Preheat the oven to 375°F/190°C/Gas 5. Line a baking sheet with parchment (baking) paper.

2 Mix all the ingredients together in a bowl. Using your hands, roll the mixture into 10 even-sized balls and place them on the prepared baking sheet, spacing them about ½ inch (1 cm) apart.

3 Turn the oven temperature down to 325°F/160°C/Gas 3 and bake the macaroons for 10–15 minutes until the edges are golden brown. Let cool on the baking sheet before enjoying. The macaroons can be stored in an airtight container for up to 7 days in the refrigerator.

4 egg whites

1 teaspoon pure vanilla powder

2 tablespoons erythritol or honey (optional—the coconut is already quite sweet)

2 cups (120 g) unsweetened desiccated coconut

Makes 10 macaroons

Per macaroon: 98 kcals, 8.7 g fat (7.5 g saturates), 0.9 g carbohydrate (0.9 g sugars), 2.2 g protein, 3 g fiber, 0.1 g salt

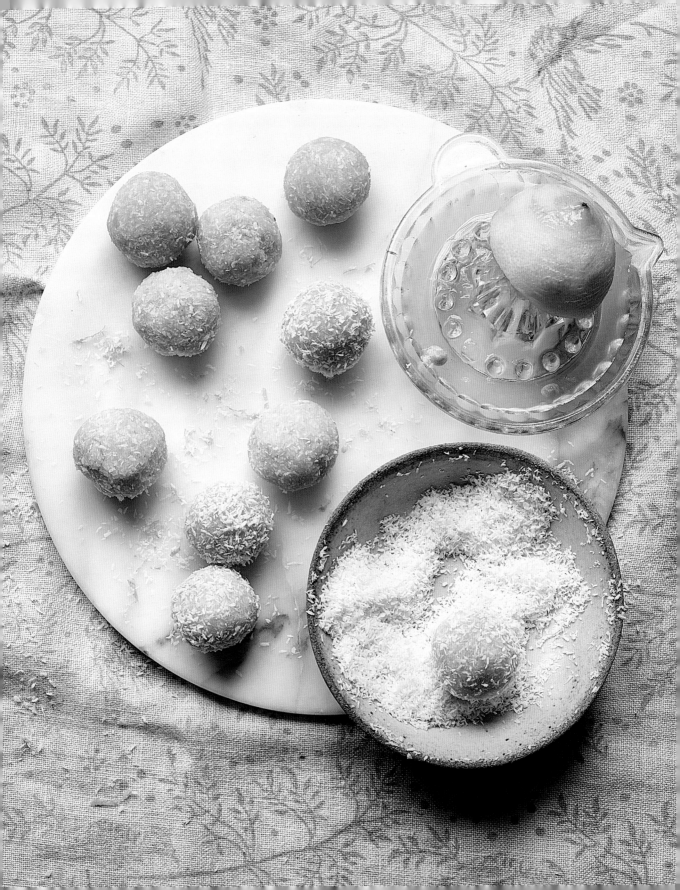

Heisse Liebe (Hot Love)

1½ cups (250 g) frozen raspberries

2 generous scoops sugar-free vanilla ice cream

Fresh mint leaves, to decorate (optional)

Serves 2

This is a great dessert that was inspired by lovers. The hot raspberry sauce melts the vanilla ice cream, reminding us how love breaks down all barriers.

1 Put the raspberries in a microwavable bowl, place the bowl in the microwave, and cook for 1 minute. Alternatively, put the raspberries in a small saucepan and cook over high heat for 1–2 minutes. Stir gently so the raspberries don't turn into mush.

2 Scoop the ice cream into chilled glasses. Pour the hot raspberry sauce over the ice cream and decorate with fresh mint leaves, if liked. Serve immediately.

Per serving: 192 kcals, 8.5 g fat (2.4 g saturates), 17.5 g carbohydrate (7.4 g sugars), 4.2 g protein, 12.1 g fiber, trace salt

Chocolate Lava Cake

This cake is quick to make, doesn't contain any flour, and is blood-sugar friendly. It's the perfect dessert to tie together a special meal. Erythritol is a natural sweetener that can be used as a substitute for sugar.

½ teaspoon butter, for greasing

2 tablespoons raw cacao powder

1–2 tablespoons erythritol

1 egg

1 tablespoon heavy whipping cream

½ teaspoon pure vanilla powder

Pinch of salt

½ teaspoon baking powder

1 Grease a coffee cup or ramekin with butter.

2 Combine the cacao powder and erythritol in a bowl, whisking to remove any lumps.

3 In a separate bowl, beat the egg until it is slightly fluffy.

4 Gently stir the beaten egg, cream, and vanilla powder into the cacao mixture. Add the salt and baking powder and mix well.

5 Pour the batter into the prepared cup or ramekin. Place the cup or ramekin in the microwave and cook for 1 minute. Check the cake for doneness: If the cake is not set and the surface is still jiggly, cook for an additional 10 seconds and then check again. Repeat until the cake is ready.

6 Serve the cake with a dollop of whipped cream and a sprinkling of cinnamon.

TO SERVE

1 tablespoon whipped cream

Ground cinnamon, for sprinkling

Serves 1

Per serving: 370 kcals, 30.6 g fat (17.3 g saturates), 4.4 g carbohydrate (0.5 g sugars), 13.2 g protein, 10.2 g fiber, 1.4 g salt

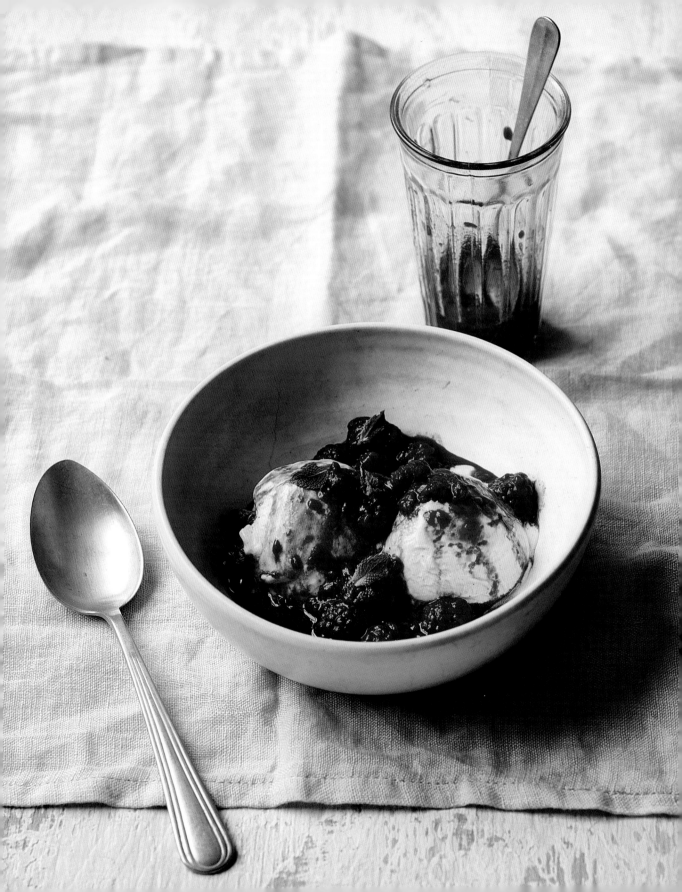

Poached Pears with Whipped Cream

Pears are delicious, particularly in the fall and winter, and can easily be found in most food markets. This dessert is healthy and looks so yummy.

1 In a saucepan large enough to hold the pears snugly, pour in the wine and lemon juice, then add the stevia, vanilla seeds or extract, cinnamon, and cloves. Squeeze the juice from the orange quarters into the saucepan, then add one of the squeezed orange quarters to the saucepan and discard the remainder. Finally, add the pears.

2 Set the saucepan over high heat and bring to a boil. Reduce the heat and simmer, uncovered, for 25 minutes, turning the pears occasionally, until they're easily pierced with the tip of a knife. Using a slotted spoon, transfer the pears to individual plates.

3 Pour the poaching liquid through a strainer set over a bowl and discard the orange quarter and spices. Return the poaching liquid to the saucepan, bring to a simmer, and cook for about 15 minutes, or until the poaching liquid is syrupy and reduced by two-thirds. Let cool a little (you don't want the syrup to melt the whipped cream).

4 Spoon the syrup over the pears and serve with the whipped cream.

Per serving: 239 kcals, 10.3 g fat (6.3 g saturates), 16.9 g carbohydrate (16.7 g sugars), 1.3 g protein, 3.6 g fiber, trace salt

1¹/₂ cups (350 ml) red wine

Juice of 1 lemon

¹/₂ teaspoon stevia

¹/₂ vanilla bean (pod), split in half lengthwise and seeds scraped out, or ¹/₄ teaspoon vanilla extract

1 cinnamon stick

5 cloves

1 orange, quartered

4 small ripe pears, peeled

Scant ¹/₂ cup (100 ml) whipping cream, whipped, to serve

Serves 4

Yeasted Popcorn

1¹/₂ tablespoons coconut oil or canola (rapeseed) oil

¹/₂ cup (90 g) popcorn kernels

1 teaspoon salt

1–2 tablespoons nutritional yeast

Serves 4

Kick your popcorn up a notch with a few shakes of nutritional yeast, which is a yellow powder that is full of B-vitamins and protein. It is vegan too! One three-cup (25-g) portion of popped popcorn counts as one serving of carbohydrate.

1 Heat the oil in a large saucepan until it melts. Add a few test popcorn kernels to the saucepan, cover, and let the kernels pop. Once the test kernels pop, add the remaining kernels. Cover the pot again and let them pop, shaking the saucepan continuously until the popping sounds subside. Turn the heat off and continue to shake the saucepan for a few more seconds.

2 Pour the popcorn into a bowl, then add the salt and nutritional yeast and stir well to mix.

Per serving: 168 kcals, 9.3 g fat (0.9 g saturates), 14.3 g carbohydrate (0.7 g sugars), 5.2 g protein, 2.8 g fiber, 1.3 g salt

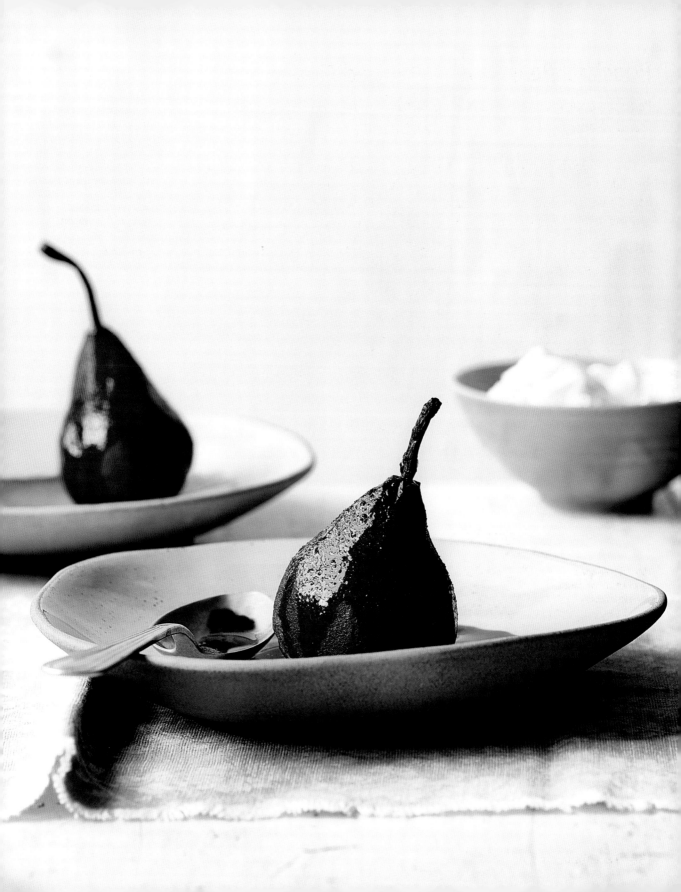

A Three-course Meal

Living with diabetes does not need to limit you when holding a dinner party. Here is a three-course meal designed by celebrated chef Antoine Camin, who is the executive chef and partner at Orsay restaurant and La Goulue of New York City. Chef Camin was instrumental in La Goulue being awarded one Michelin star in the famous Guide Michelin. I have had the privilege of knowing Chef Camin for almost five years, and when I asked him for some recipes that would be suitable for a person living with diabetes, he gladly provided a delicious menu that everyone can enjoy.

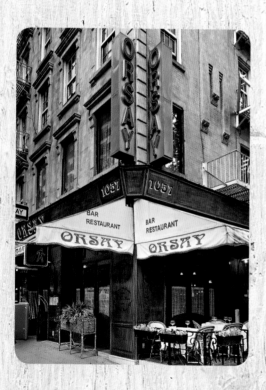

SALMON TARTARE WITH TROUT CAVIAR

1 x 1-lb (450-g) skinless wild salmon fillet

½ cup (120 g) trout caviar, plus extra to garnish

¼ cup (60 ml) olive oil

2 tablespoons soy sauce

2 tablespoons lime juice

10 shiso leaves (also known as perilla leaves), chopped, plus 4 whole leaves, to garnish

2 scallions (spring onions), chopped

Scant ½ teaspoon (2 g) wasabi paste

½ teaspoon cayenne pepper

Salt and freshly ground black pepper

Tortilla or crispy rice chips, to serve (optional)

Serves 4

1 Chop the salmon into ¼-inch (5-mm cubes), then put in a bowl set over another larger bowl of ice to chill.

2 Once the salmon has chilled, add the remaining ingredients, and gently mix together with a spoon—you need to do this gently to prevent the fish eggs from popping. Season to taste with salt and pepper.

3 Divide among small chilled bowls and garnish each portion with a whole shiso leaf and a teaspoon of caviar. Serve with tortilla or crispy rice chips, if liked.

Per serving: 408 kcals, 29.4 g fat (5.4 g saturates), 3.2 g carbohydrate (1.8 g sugars), 32.8 g protein, 0.1 g fiber, 2.6 g salt

DORADE WITH SUN-DRIED TOMATO SALSA

Pinch of kosher salt

6 yellow-fleshed potatoes, rinsed

4 dorade (sea bream) fillets, about 6 oz (175 g)

1¹/₂ teaspoons Espelette pepper (piment d'Espelette)

6 tablespoons extra virgin olive oil, divided

Fennel fronds, to garnish

FOR THE SALSA

3 cups (175 g) sun-dried tomatoes, diced

10 marinated white anchovies, diced

6 tablespoons extra virgin olive oil

2 tablespoons pitted Niçoise olives, diced

2 tablespoons pine nuts

2 tablespoons capers

Juice of ¹/₂ lemon

Salt and freshly ground black pepper

Serves 4

Per serving: 972 kcals, 50 g fat (6.2 g saturates), 75 g carbohydrate (20.4 g sugars), 48 g protein, 12.5 g fiber, 2.1 g salt

1 Preheat the oven to 400°F/ 200°C/Gas 6. Spread a layer of kosher salt over the bottom of a roasting pan.

2 Arrange the potatoes on top of the salt and bake for 45 minutes, or until soft. Once the potatoes are cool enough to handle, remove the skins and use a fork to roughly crush the flesh in a bowl. Set aside.

3 Prepare the salsa by combining all the ingredients in a bowl. Taste, and adjust the seasoning if necessary.

4 Cut the fish fillets in half and season with salt and Espelette pepper. Heat 1 tablespoon of the oil in a nonstick skillet (frying pan) over medium heat, add the fish, skin-side down, and cook for about 7 minutes, or until cooked through.

5 Just before you are ready to serve, season the crushed potatoes with salt and pepper, then stir in the remaining oil.

6 To serve, spoon the crushed potatoes into the center of each plate, top with 2 pieces of fish and a generous serving of the salsa, and garnish with some fennel fronds.

HONEY AND FRUIT PANNA COTTAS

2¹/₂ silver gelatin leaves

¹/₂ cup (120 ml) milk

3 tablespoons honey

Grated zest of ¹/₂ lemon

Grated zest of ¹/₂ orange

¹/₂ teaspoon vanilla paste (purée)

3 saffron threads

1³/₄ cups (300 ml) heavy (double) cream

¹/₃ cup (50 g) strawberries, quartered

¹/₃ cup (50 g) raspberries

¹/₃ cup (50 g) blueberries

Serves 4

Per serving: 415 kcals, 36.6 g fat (22.7 g saturates), 16.9 g carbohydrate (16.8 g sugars), 2.8 g protein, 1.4 g fiber, 0.1 g salt

1 Soak the gelatin in a little cold water for a few minutes, then squeeze it dry.

2 Meanwhile, pour the milk into a saucepan, add the honey, lemon and orange zest, vanilla paste (purée), and saffron and bring to a boil. Remove from the heat and set aside until the mixture has cooled a little but is still hot. Add the gelatin and stir until it has completely dissolved. Pour in the heavy (double) cream and mix well, then let sit for 2 hours at room temperature to let the flavors infuse.

3 Strain the mixture through a fine strainer (sieve) into a pitcher or clean bowl, then pour into 4 glasses. Chill in the refrigerator for 2–3 hours until set.

4 To make the berry compote, place all the berries in a small saucepan and cook over low heat until the berries start to simmer. Remove from the heat and let cool.

5 When you are ready to serve, garnish the panna cottas with the compote.

Conclusion: Fears and Hopes

For a person living with a serious chronic disease, every day is a new fight. Getting up each morning involves motivating oneself to stick to treatment schedules, diets, and routines. Sometimes this can feel unfair, like a huge, almost overwhelming struggle. It may seem easier to just stop fighting and let go, but that is not an option for those with most chronic conditions, because late-stage complications are often the result of poor management of the disease. In the case of T1D, the complications are, in many cases, worse than the disease itself.

Receiving my diagnosis

I know the sense of helplessness and futility that comes from living with a chronic disease. When I first received a diagnosis of T1D, I saw my condition as a failure—something I had never fully experienced before. Sure, I had lost tennis matches and made mistakes in school tests, but when it came down to it, I had not really failed at anything I cared about. My parents loved me, and my sisters were my close friends. I never felt alone. Yet, the day I got my diagnosis, I felt utterly alone.

In my early years with diabetes, I never allowed the disease to be a part of me. I vowed it would not hinder nor stop me, nor make me seem weaker or different. I viewed the world through the eyes of a teenager. I did not have the maturity to understand that everyone has something they are not proud of—ranging from asthma to alcoholism to just having an awkward-looking nose. We all suffer through some indignity that makes us self-conscious, and we must learn to cope with those perceived flaws.

Still, the psychological aspects of realizing one has diabetes can impact people very differently. In my case, I chose to learn everything I could about the medical and scientific aspects of the disease—to the extent that I obtained an MD and a PhD, followed by post-doc work at the Joslin Diabetes Center at Harvard Medical School, and then fifteen years in industry and on Wall Street learning about the business of diabetes.

This commitment to overachievement in every area of my life was part of my plan to overcome this physical failure. I had made a promise to myself that I was not going to let diabetes change me and that I was going to show everyone that I could be better at the things I set out to do than people who did not have a disability. It was a tough task and a very tiresome way of living. Fighting every moment and trying to prove oneself makes for a stressful, very lonely existence. Instead of asking for help or using my vulnerability to get sympathy or love, I chose the opposite. I elected to dismiss anyone who wanted to get close to me or treated me differently.

Hiding my diabetes

To avoid the shame of feeling inferior, I decided to keep my diabetes a secret. So during my first ten years with T1D, I took hiding my disease to the extreme, so much so that my teachers and colleagues in the Department of Diabetology at the Karolinska Institutet and at the Joslin Diabetes Center had no clue I had diabetes. I studied the disease thoroughly, discussed it daily, and examined diabetic patients, all while hiding my own affliction. I had a deep shame and even contempt for the diabetes inside of me, and I never really acknowledged that it was a part of me.

I kept my diabetes under tight control and requested that my family stay quiet about my condition. They agreed to live with my secret, which only exacerbated my feeling of being a failure and defective. I do not blame my parents or sisters at all, since they could not know what I was going through, and they did not dare to speak openly about the issues facing our family, since I was so strongly against disclosing the truth. Luckily for us, I was very healthy during this time and did not need much extra care beyond the psychological help that I had so emphatically dismissed.

This behavior caused some problems, of course, since I could not ask for help, and some of my actions were difficult to

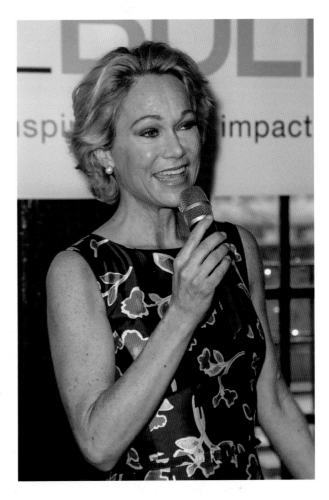

One of the goals of my organization, Lyfebulb, is to connect people, both those with disease and those who care for someone with disease

explain. When I suffered from a low blood sugar episode, I had to run off to the bathroom where I would stuff my face with sugary drinks or fruit that I kept stashed in my purse. If I were unprepared, I had to quickly buy and ingest something, hiding my behavior until I evened out. When I declined desserts and snacks people kindly offered, it was always a defensive move on my part. I began to realize I came across as rude or even as someone with an eating disorder. My reaction was harsh because I did not know how to explain my

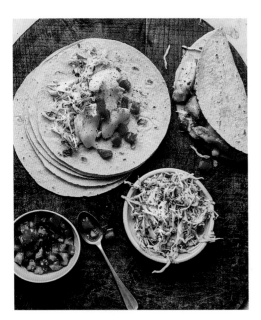

A healthier life includes a healthier diet—and you can start by using the recipes provided. These are the Fish Tacos with Herby Slaw on page 114.

rejection each time. And having grown up in a family where I had been taught to finish my meals and always taste a little of what was offered, I felt impolite when I kept declining sweets or leaving large portions of food on my plate. Meals and social occasions became stressful for me, and that affected my behavior even more. Because I anticipated having to deal with these issues in social settings, I became somewhat highly strung.

Living in denial

This period of super-control ended dramatically when I had finished my education in Sweden and went to Harvard University for my post-doc. I stopped being obsessed with my sugars, and like an overweight person who doesn't like to step on the scale, I stopped measuring my glucose levels. I knew my sugars were high, but I did not care anymore. I just wanted to be normal, and as a twenty-five-year-old double doctor (physician and PhD), I started to let loose. In medical school I had had two very serious relationships, each lasting three years. Probably either could have led to marriage and children if I had elected to stick with them. In Boston I was reliving my teenage years and went on many dates. Instead of thinking about the future and fighting to stay free of complications, I started living in the moment. It was so much easier.

I think this is a common reaction of people living with chronic disease. When you are told that your disease may trigger blindness, kidney failure, or amputations of your feet and legs, and when you have seen this happen to patients on a daily basis (which I had as a young doctor), you have to make a choice. You can accept all the help you can get, you can fight the disease without help from others, or you can just go with the flow and live in the moment. I was young, attractive, and in the best environment in the world for the kind of work I wanted to pursue. I spent the next ten years throwing myself at challenging opportunities, competing for top jobs, and engaging in relationships that I knew were never going to make it in the long term. It felt safe, and, after all, I never expected to live well into old age. I was sure something would happen that would eliminate my risk of suffering as an older sick person, so why not just live in the present? Above all, such carefree behavior meant I would not need to open up fully and ask for help.

Unfortunately, diabetes is not something you can take a vacation from or simply ignore. It was not until eighteen years post diagnosis—when my world came falling down due to kidney and eye complications—that I was forced to discuss my diabetes with colleagues and friends. In frail health and knowing I needed a kidney transplant to save my life, I finally admitted to myself and others that I had a debilitating disease. But even then, I felt uncomfortable doing so and still could not accept the disease as my own. In fact, I simply felt tired, and I wanted to die.

But then something happened that changed my attitude. As I was facing death, I saw the pain in my parents' eyes and heard the frustration in my friends' voices. I realized I had to fight, but this time out in the open. I did my research and found the best possible treatment pathway, and I was fortunate enough to have incredible support in my parents and friends. After both a kidney transplant and a pancreas transplant, my body was somewhat repaired; now I could move on to the task of repairing my mind. The process of going through the transplants is the content of a separate book, since it involves such complexity from a medical and emotional angle.

A world of opportunity

The ultimate advice I can provide to others living with diabetes is to accept and take responsibility of your own disease while allowing others to help you and learn from you about diabetes. For years I hated the word "diabetes," and I know many other people who live with the disease feel as I did. That is why we use other ways to refer to someone who has diabetes, because having the disease does not mean you are defined solely by the disease. However, it also does not mean you can deny that diabetes is part of you.

So, instead of seeing diabetes as a negative, you can choose to view it as an opportunity to develop habits that support a healthier life, to be more aware of and disciplined about maintaining good health in general, and to educate and help others improve their own health and physical condition, i.e., living by example and even mentoring. If you are entrepreneurial in your mindset, diabetes could give you a reason to pursue a path toward a career in developing new solutions that could help yourself and others. It is up to us, people living with diabetes, to educate the masses—those who do not understand what diabetes does to the body, what restrictions we face and opportunities we have, and how they can best help us. Doctors and scientists can lecture about the medical science of diabetes, but they cannot feel the disease the way we can. They have no way of knowing what a low blood sugar really does to our bodies and minds and how severe high blood sugar makes us feel groggy and slow. It is so important for those of us with this disease to get involved at various levels in society to improve the care and the instruments available to people with diabetes.

For those with diabetes, speaking publicly about the disease is important so that our society realizes how difficult it is to live with the disease

Advocates for people afflicted with other diseases, such as cancer or HIV/AIDS, have been very vocal about the threats, the suffering, and the perception of that disease in society. Diabetes, however, has not achieved such a high profile nor received adequate media attention and, frankly, the "average" person knows little about its causes and debilitating effects. Diabetes is not a disease we have caused ourselves, it is not something we ate ourselves into, and it is not the disease of lazy people who live on junk food and can't get up off the couch. As I mentioned earlier on in this book, T1D and T2D have different etiologies and are caused by multiple factors. However, we can benefit from identifying them earlier and, hopefully in the future, preventing them outright.

Making a difference

For those with diabetes, speaking publicly about the disease is important so that our society realizes how difficult it is to live with the disease and companies can become inspired to start working harder on cures and better treatments. I have never encountered an individual who has not been moved to tears when listening to a young child relate how his or her days are regulated by injections and monitoring, or hearing parents voice their fears when their young child is away from them and they cannot control the highs and the lows. For people with T1D, only one drug (and its variations) has been available since 1921: insulin. Insulin saves lives and makes people with T1D productive individuals in society if they manage their disease correctly, but how is it possible that there have been no transformative medical advancements in this area in almost a hundred years? There must be something better!

I hope that stories like mine can inspire people to change, and I hope to affect lives for the better

Healthcare professionals often perceive the disease to be difficult to manage by prescribing drugs only, and since few procedures are involved, but rather mostly education, physicians do not get paid well for managing diabetes patients, nor do they get bonuses if their patients are managed better. Diabetes patients on average are notoriously noncompliant, which means they do not take their drugs the way they should or prick their fingers to measure blood glucose often enough. This is somewhat understandable, as living with diabetes stinks; most diabetics find constantly monitoring their disease to be tedious, which explains why patients sometimes just want to escape from those demands. But when we do that, we punish and cripple ourselves.

We need to structure the system differently, so that doctors and nurses are incentivized to help us get back on track, and to add the "force amplifier"—that being "patients helping patients"—by creating mentoring programs where people with more experience can teach those who are new to the demands of diabetes or who find themselves slipping. Trust of a fellow patient is higher than trust for a doctor who doesn't have the disease. These programs will also lessen the burden for the doctors and allow them to focus on items that actually require medical expertise rather than experience in living with the disease.

Stimulating young scientists to develop new technologies and drugs, perhaps even starting companies and increasing funding for these companies, is critical for the future of diabetes care. I have already mentioned patient entrepreneurs, but we must also provide companies that venture into this space with incentives. Regulatory pathways must be expedited and the time to market lessened so that venture investors place bets on small companies, allowing them to compete with the larger companies that are so heavily entrenched in the existing markets.

In summary, I believe we as players in the diabetes ecosystem must empower diabetes patients but also place full accountability on them to be the leaders in this fight against a global pandemic that is crippling our people and our economy. By developing mentoring programs, organizing events where speakers can present information on the subject, and creating venues for patient entrepreneurs, we give patients important roles in this fight. By educating society, the medical community, and industry, we change the perception of the disease and create solutions to fight the battle.

Looking toward my future

As I write this, it has been six years since the kidney transplant and five years of being off insulin, thanks to the new pancreas. I am now beginning to believe in a future. I still wake up every day with

Instead of seeing diabetes as a negative, you can choose to view it as an opportunity to develop habits that support a healthier life, to be more aware of and disciplined about maintaining good health in general, and to educate and help others improve their own health

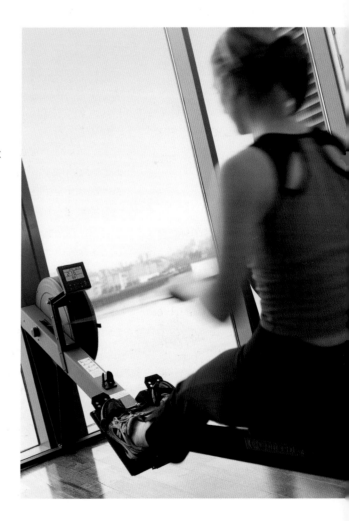

> I am learning to trust people to be there for me and that I am not alone, and I am beginning to believe I can be happy and that I can help other people be happy

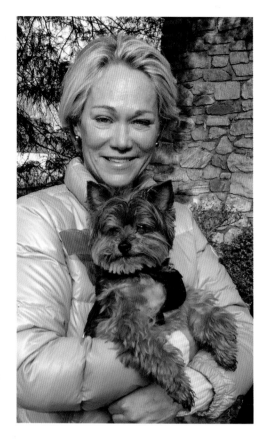

a mindset of needing to fight to stay alive, but I am learning to trust people to be there for me and that I am not alone. I am beginning to believe I can be happy and that I can help other people be happy. However, it is hard to live for a future after so many years. Each time I have to fight for my health again, I wonder what the purpose is. It would be easier to just give up. And then I think about the people around me who love me and believe in me, and I cannot give up. I have to fight beyond today, try to live more patiently, and be less concerned about completing every task as fast as possible, as if there were no tomorrow.

One of the goals for my new venture, Lyfebulb, is to connect people, both those with disease and those who care for someone with disease, and allow for everything from small daily struggles to major issues to be discussed and solved through improved funding, more targeted research, and better access to care. I hope that stories like mine can inspire people to change, and I hope to affect lives for the better. I have learned to see the positives in darkness and to seek highs when there are mostly lows. Now is the time for me to search for some steadiness and, above all, to believe in my own future.

Useful Resources

Organizations for People with Diabetes

USA

Academy of Nutrition and Dietetics
120 South Riverside Plaza
Suite 2000
Chicago, IL 60606-6995
eatright.org

American Association of Clinical Endocrinologists (AACE)
245 Riverside Avenue
Suite 200
Jacksonville, FL 32202
aace.com

American Association of Diabetes Educators (AADE)
200 West Madison Street
Suite 800
Chicago, IL 60606
diabeteseducator.org

American Diabetes Association
1701 North Beauregard Street
Alexandria, VA 22311
www.diabetes.org

Centers for Disease Control and Prevention (CDC)
Division of Diabetes
1600 Clifton Road
Atlanta, GA 30329-4027
cdc.gov/diabetes

Children's Diabetes Foundation
4380 S Syracuse Street
Suite 430
Denver, CO 80237
childrensdiabetesfoundation.org

Children with Diabetes
8216 Princeton-Glendale
Road, PMB 200
West Chester
OH 45069-1675
childrenwithdiabetes.com

Close Concerns
804 Haight Street
San Francisco, CA 94117
closeconcerns.com

Diabetes Action
6701 Democracy Boulevard
Suite 300
Bethesda, MD 20817
diabetesaction.org

Diabetes Care and Education (DCE)
www.dce.org

Diabetes Community Advocacy Foundation
diabetescaf.org

Diabetes Hands Foundation
1962 University Ave, #1
Berkeley, CA 94704
diabeteshandsfoundation.org

dLife
101 Franklin Street
Westport, CT 06880
dlife.com

Endocrine Society
2055 L Street NW
Suite 600
Washington, DC 20036
endocrine.org

Glu
T1D Exchange
11 Avenue de Lafayette
5th Floor
Boston, MA 02111
t1dexchange.org

Indian Health Service (IHS)
Division of Diabetes
Treatment and Prevention
5600 Fishers Lane
Rockville, MD 20857
ihs.gov/medicalprograms/diabetes

The International Society on Hypertension in Blacks (ISHIB)
2111 Wilson Boulevard
Suite 700
Arlington, VA 22201
ishib.org

Juvenile Diabetes Research Foundation (JDRF)
26 Broadway, 14th floor
New York, NY 10004
jdrf.org

National Eye Institute (NEI)
31 Center Drive, MSC 2510
Bethesda, MD 20892-2510
nei.nih.gov

National Institute of Diabetes and Digestive and Kidney Disease
9000 Rockville Pike
Bethesda, MD 20892-2560
niddk.nih.gov

National Kidney Foundation
30 East 33rd Street
New York, NY 10016
kidney.org

Nephrogenic Diabetes Insipidus Foundation (NDIF)
Main Street, PO Box 1390
Eastsound, WA 98245
ndif.org

United States Department of Veterans Affairs
Office of Specialty Care
Services
810 Vermont Avenue NW
Washington, DC 20420
va.gov/diabetes/#veterans

CANADA

Canadian Diabetes Association
diabetes.ca

Diabetes Hope Foundation
6150 Dixie Road, Unit #1
Mississauga, Ontario L5T 2E2
diabeteshopefoundation.com

Diabetes Québec
8550 Pie-IX Boulevard
Suite 300
Montréal, Québec H1Z4G2
diabete.qc.ca

Juvenile Diabetes Research Foundation (JDRF)
jdrf.ca

The National Aborginal Diabetes Association
103–90 Garry Street
Winnipeg, Manitoba
R3C 4H1
nada.ca

UK

Beating Diabetes
beatingdiabetes.org

Black and Ethnic Minority Diabetes Association (BEMDA)
St. Paul's Church Centre
Rossmore Road
London NW1 6NJ
bemda.org

The British Journal of Diabetes
bjdvd.com

British Society for Paediatric Endocrinology and Diabetes
c/o BioScientifica Ltd
Euro House, 22 Apex Court
Woodlands, Bristol BS32 4JT
bsped.org.uk

Diabetes Research Network
Diabetes Research Network
Coordinating Centre
ICCH Building
Imperial College
59–61 North Wharf Road
London W2 1LA
ukdrn.org

Diabetes UK
Macleod House, 10 Parkway
London NW1 7AA
diabetes.org.uk

Diabetes Research and Wellness Foundation (DRWF)
010-012 Northney Marina
Hayling Island, Hampshire
PO11 0NH
drwf.org.uk

The Diabetic Foot
diabeticfoot.org.uk

InDependent Diabetes Trust (IDDT)
PO Box 294
Northampton NN1 4XS
iddt.org

Juvenile Diabetes Research Institute (JDRF)
jdrf.org.uk

Leicestershire Diabetes
leicestershirediabetes.org.uk

AUSTRALIA

Australian Diabetes Educators Association (ADEA)
Unit 6, 70 Maclaurin Crescent
Chifley, ACT 2606
adea.com.au

Australian Diabetes in Pregnancy Society
145 Macquarie Street
Sydney, NSW 2000
adips.org

Australian Diabetes Society (ADS)
145 Macquarie Street
Sydney, NSW 2000
diabetessociety.com.au

Australasian Paediatric Endocrine Group
PO Box 180
Morisset, NSW 2264
apeg.org.au

Baker IDI Heart and Diabetes Institute
75 Commercial Road
Melbourne, VIC 3004
bakeridi.edu.au

Diabetes Australia
Level 1, 101 Northbourne Ave
Turner, ACT 2612
diabetesaustralia.com.au

Diabetes Research Western Australia
PO Box X2213
Perth, WA 6847
diabetesresearchwa.com.au

Juvenile Diabetes Research Foundation (JDRF)
jdrf.org.au

Stop Diabetes Australia
stopdiabetes.com.au

NEW ZEALAND

Diabetes New Zealand
Level 7, 15 Murphy Street
PO Box 12441
Thorndon, Wellington
diabetes.org.nz

Diabetes NZ Auckland Branch
Level 2, 92–94 Beachcroft
Avenue Onehunga
Auckland 1061
diabetesauckland.org.nz

Diabetes Youth New Zealand
PO Box 56172,
Dominion Road
Auckland 1446
diabetesyouth.org.nz

New Zealand Society for the Study of Diabetes (NZSSD)
c/o Edgar National Centre
for Diabetes Research
Department of Medicine
University of Otago
PO Box 56
Dunedin 9054
nzssd.org.nz

SOUTH AFRICA

Diabetes South Africa
PO Box 7828
Roggebaai, Cape Town, 8012
diabetessa.org.za

South African Diabetes Association (SADA)
home.intekom.com/
buildlink/ips/sada

Sweet Life
PO Box 12651, Mill Street
Western Cape, 8010
sweetlifemag.co.za

Major Academic Institutions Working in Diabetes

USA

Albert Einstein College of Medicine
1300 Morris Park Avenue
Bronx, NY 10461
einstein.yu.edu/centers/
diabetes-research

Barbara Davis Center for Childhood Diabetes
1775 Aurora Court
Aurora, CO 80045
ucdenver.edu/academics/
colleges/medicalschool/
centers/BarbaraDavis

Baylor College of Medicine, Diabetes Research Center
Alkek Building for Biomedical
Research, Room 618
One Baylor Plaza, BCM185
Houston, TX 77030
bcm.edu/diabetescenter

Boston Area Diabetes Endocrinology Research Center (BADERC)
baderc.org

Columbia University, Diabetes Research Center
Russ Berrie Medical
Sciences Pavilion
1150 Nicholas Avenue
Suite 238
New York, NY 10032
derc.cumc.columbia.edu/
index.php

Diabetes Research Centers
diabetescenters.org

Johns Hopkins University-University of Maryland, Diabetes Research Center
600 North Wolfe Street
CMSC 10–113
Baltimore, MD 21287
hopkinsmedicine.org/drtc

Joslin Diabetes Center and Joslin Clinic
One Joslin Place
Boston, MA 02215
joslin.org

UCSD-UCLA, Diabetes Research Center
derc.ucsd.edu

UCSF, Diabetes Center
513 Parnassus Avenue
Room 1116
San Francisco, CA 94143
diabetes.ucsf.edu/contact-us

University of Alabama at Birmingham, Diabetes Research Center
616 Webb Nutrition
Sciences Building
1675 University Boulevard
Birmingham, AL 35294-3360
uab.edu/shp/drc/

University of Chicago, Diabetes Research and Training Center (DRTC)
5841 South Maryland
Avenue, AMB N237, MC1207
Chicago, IL 60637
drtc.bsd.uchicago.edu

University of Michigan, Diabetes Research Center and Center for Diabetes Translational Research
Brehm Tower
1000 Wall Street
Ann Arbor, MI 48105
diabetesresearch.med.umich.
edu

University of Pennsylvania, Diabetes Research Center
3400 Civic Center Boulevard
Philadelphia, PA 19104-5160
med.upenn.edu/idom/derc

University of Washington, Diabetes Research Center
1660 South Columbian Way
Seattle, WA 98108-1597
depts.washington.edu/
diabetes

Vanderbilt University, Diabetes Center and Diabetes Research and Training Center
2215 Garland Avenue
Nashville, TN 37232
mc.vanderbilt.edu/diabetes/
drtc

Washington University in St Louis, School of Medicine Diabetes Research Center
660 South Euclid Avenue
St. Louis, MO 63110
diabetesresearchcenter.dom.
wustl.edu

Yale School of Medicine, Diabetes Research Center
300 Cedar Street, TAC S141
New Haven, CT 06520-8020
derc.yale.edu/index.aspx

CANADA

Alberta Diabetes Institute, University of Alberta
1-002 Li Ka Shing Centre for
Health Research Innovation
Edmonton, Alberta T6G 2E1
adi.ualberta.ca

Banting and Best Diabetes Centre, University of Toronto
Eaton Building, 12th Floor
Room 12E248
Toronto General Hospital,
200 Elizabeth Street
Toronto, Ontario M5G 2C4
bbdc.org

Lawson Health Research Institute
750 Base Line Road East
Suite 300
London, Ontario N6C2R5
lawsonresearch.ca

Lunenfeld-Tanenbaum Research Institute
982–600 University Avenue
Toronto, Ontario M5G 1X5
lunenfeld.ca

UK

Diabetes Research Network Coordinating Centre
ICCH Building
Imperial College
59–61 North Wharf Road
London W2 1LA
ukdrn.org

Diabetes Research Unit Cymru
Institute of Life Science
3rd Floor
Singleton Park, Swansea
SA2 8PP
diabeteswales.org.uk

Imperial College London, Division of Diabetes, Endocrinology and Metabolism
Level 2, Faculty Building
South Kensington Campus
London SW7 2AZ
imperial.ac.uk

National Institute for Health Research
crn.nihr.ac.uk/diabetes/

Newcastle University, Diabetes Research Group
Faculty of Medical Sciences,
The Medical School
Framlington Place
Newcastle upon Tyne
NE2 4HH
ncl.ac.uk/medicalsciences/
research/groups/diabetes

NHS Research Scotland
The Golden Jubilee National
Hospital, Level 4 East
Agamemnon Street
Clydebank G81 4DY
nhsresearchscotland.org.uk/
research-areas/diabetes

Northern Ireland Clinical Research Network (NICRN)
NICRN Co-ordinating Centre
Room 2007, 2nd Floor
King Edward Building
The Royal Hospitals
Grosvenor Road
Belfast BT12 6BA
nicrn.hscni.net

Scottish Diabetes Research Network (SDRN) Diabetes Support Unit
Level 8
Ninewells Hospital
Dundee DD1 9SY
sdrn.org.uk

University of Cambridge, School of Clinical Medicine
Hills Road
Cambridge CB2 0SP
medschl.cam.ac.uk/research

University of Glasgow, Institute of Cardiovasular and Medical Sciences, Metabolic Disease and Diabetes Research
Glasgow G12 8QQ
gla.ac.uk/researchinstitutes/
icams/research/metabolic
diseasediabetesresearch

University of Leicester, Diabetes Research Centre
Leicester General Hospital
Leicester LE5 4PW
le.ac.uk/colleges/
medbiopsych/research/drc

The University of Manchester, Centre for Endocrinology and Diabetes
AV Hill Building, Oxford Road
Manchester M13 9PT
human-development.
manchester.ac.uk/
endocrinologyanddiabetes

University of Oxford, Diabetes Trials Unit
OCDEM Building, Churchill
Hospital, Old Road
Headington, Oxford OX3 7LJ
dtu.ox.ac.uk

AUSTRALIA

Baker IDI Heart and Diabetes Institute (Alice Springs)
W & E Rubuntja Building
Alice Springs Hospital
Campus, Gap Road
Alice Springs, NT 0870
bakeridi.edu.au

Baker IDI Heart and Diabetes Institute (Melbourne)
75 Commercial Road
Melbourne, VIC 3004
bakeridi.edu.au

Diabetes Research Western Australia
PO Box X2213
Perth, WA 6847
diabetesresearchwa.com.au

Flinders University
Sturt Road
Bedford Park, SA 5042
flinders.edu.au

Garvan Institute of Medical Research
384 Victoria Street
Darlinghurst, Sydney, NSW 2010
garvan.org.au

The University of Adelaide
Adelaide, SA 5005
adelaide.edu.au

NEW ZEALAND

The Diabetes Research Institute
Don Beavan Medical
Research Centre 2/40
Stewart Street
Christchurch 8011
diabetesresearchinstitutetrust.
co.nz

Edgar Diabetes and Obesity Research
Dunedin School of Medicine,
University of Otago
PO Box 56
Dunedin 9054
otago.ac.nz/diabetes/index.
html

Health Research Council of New Zealand
50 Grafton Road
Grafton, Auckland 1010
hrc.govt.nz

Liggins Institute, University of Auckland
Private Bag 92019
Auckland 1142
liggins.auckland.ac.nz/en/
for/thecommunity/gems-
study.html

SOUTH AFRICA

Chronic Disease Initiative for Africa
J47/86 Old Main Building
Groote Schuur Hospital
Observatory
Cape Town, 7925
cdia.uct.ac.za

University of KwaZulu-Natal, Department of Diabetes and Endocrinology, School of Clinical Medicine
719 Umbilo Road
Congella, 4013
endocrinology.ukzn.ac.za

Stellenbosch University
Private Bag X1
Matieland, Stellenbosch, 7602
sun.ac.za/english

Blogs and Websites

Lyfebulb (Karin's organization)
lyfebulb.com

A Sweet Life
asweetlife.org/blogs

Bitter-Sweet (Karen Graffeo)
bittersweetdiabetes.com

Diabetes Community Advocacy Foundation
diabetescaf.org

Diabetes Daily
diabetesdaily.com

Diabetes Hands Foundation
diabeteshandsfoundation.org/our-blog

Diabetes Mine
healthline.com/diabetesmine

Diabetes Self-Management
diabetesselfmanagement.com/blog

Diabetes Sisters
diabetessisters.org

Diabetes Stops Here
diabetesstopshere.org

Diabetes Stories (Riva Greenberg)
diabetesstories.com/stories blog

Diabetesaliciousness (Kelly Kunik)
diabetesaliciousness.blogspot.com

DLife
dlife.com/diabetes-blog

D-Mom (Leighann Calentine)
d-mom.com

EndocrineWeb
endocrineweb.com

Every Day Ups and Downs
everydayupsanddowns.co.uk

I Run on Insulin (Alexis Pollack)
irunoninsulin.com

Insulin Nation
insulinnation.com

Ninjabetic (George Simmons)
ninjabetic.com

Omnipod
myomnipod.com

Our Diabetic Life (Meri)
ourdiabeticlife.com

Scott's Diabetes (Scott K. Johnson)
scottsdiabetes.com

Shoot Up or Put Up (Tim Brown and Alison Finney)
shootuporputup.co.uk

Six Until Me (Kerri Sparling)
sixuntilme.com

Texting My Pancreas (Kim Vlasnik)
textingmypancreas.com

TuDiabetes
tudiabetes.org/blogs

Books on Diabetes

Becker, Gretchen. *Prediabetes: What You Need to Know to Keep Diabetes Away*, Marlowe & Company, 2004.

Bernstein, Richard K. *Dr. Bernstein's Diabetes Solution: A Complete Guide to Achieving Normal Blood Sugars*, Little, Brown and Company, 1997.

Blackstone, Margaret. *Beat Diabetes!: How I Overcame Diabetes and You Can Too!*, Adams Media Corporation, 1999.

Challem, Jack. *Stop Prediabetes Now: The Ultimate Plan to Lose Weight and Prevent Diabetes*, John Wiley & Sons, Inc., 2007.

Colberg, Sheri. *Diabetic Athlete's Handbook*, Human Kinetics, 2009.

Deutscher, Andrew. *Typecast: Amazing People Overcoming the Chronic Disease of Type 1 Diabetes*, Humbition Entertainment, 2014.

Eichten, Chuck. *The Book of Better: Life with Diabetes Can't Be Perfect. Make It Better*, Three Rivers Press, 2011.

Fuselier, Rhonda W. *Mommy Can't Fix It: Coping with Type One Diabetes*, CreateSpace Independent Publishing Platform, 2013.

Gosselin, Kim, and Freedman, Moss. *Taking Diabetes to School* (Special Kids in Schools Series), JayJo Books, 2004.

Greene, Bob. *The Best Life Guide to Managing Diabetes and Pre-Diabetes*, Simon & Schuster, 2009.

Hirsch, James S. *Cheating Destiny: Living with Diabetes*, Mariner Books, 2007.

McCarthy, Moira. *The Everything Parent's Guide To Children With Juvenile Diabetes: Reassuring Advice for Managing Symptoms and Raising a Happy, Healthy Child*, Adams Media, 2007.

Rubin, Dr Alan L. *Prediabetes For Dummies*, Wiley Publishing Inc., 2010.

Ruhl, Jenny. *Blood Sugar 101: What They Don't Tell You About Diabetes*, Technion Books, 2016.

Scalpi, Gretchen. *The Everything Guide to Managing and Reversing Pre-Diabetes: Your Complete Plan for Preventing the Onset of Diabetes*, Adams Media, 2011.

Scheiner, Gary. *Think Like a Pancreas: A Practical Guide to Managing Diabetes with Insulin*, Da Capo Press, 2011.

Sparling, Kerri. *Balancing Diabetes: Conversations About Finding Happiness and Living Well*, Spry Publishing, 2014.

Sutherland, Phil, and Hanc, John. *Not Dead Yet: My Race Against Disease: From Diagnosis to Dominance*, Thomas Dunne Books, 2011.

Walsh, John, *et al. Using Insulin: Everything You Need for Success with Insulin*, Torrey Pines Press, 2003.

Wright, Hillary. *The Prediabetes Diet Plan: How to Reverse Prediabetes and Prevent Diabetes Through Healthy Eating and Exercise*, Ten Speed Press, 2013.

Major Biopharma and Medical Device Companies Working in Diabetes

Abbott
abbott.com

AbbVie
abbvie.com

Akros Pharma
akrospharma.com

Amgen
amgen.com

AstraZeneca
astrazeneca.com

Beta-O2 Technologies
beta-o2.com

Biocon
biocon.com

BioLineRx
biolinerx.com

Boehringer Ingelheim
boehringeringelheim.com

Boston Therapeutics
bostonti.com

Bristol-Myers Squibb
bms.com

ConjuChem
conjuchem.com

Dexcom
dexcom.com

Diatranz Otsuka
dolglobal.com

DiaVacs
diavacs.us.com

Elcelyx Therapeutics
elcelyx.com

Eli Lilly and Company
lilly.com

Encapsulife
encapsulife.org

Generex Biotechnology
generex.com

Gilead
gilead.com

GlaxoSmithKline
gsk.com

Harvest Moon Pharmaceuticals
harvestmoonpharma.com

Intarcia Therapeutics
intarcia.com

Ionis Pharmaceuticals
ionispharma.com

Islet Sciences
isletsciences.com

Johnson & Johnson
jnj.com

Kadmon
kadmon.com

Lexicon Pharmaceuticals
lexpharma.com

MacroGenics
macrogenics.com

MannKind Corporation
mannkindcorp.com

Medtronic
medtronic.com

Merck
merck.com

NGM Biopharmaceuticals
ngmbio.com

Novartis
novartis.com

Novo Nordisk
novonordisk.com

Oramed Pharmaceuticals
oramed.com

Perle Bioscience
perlebioscience.com

Pfizer
pfizer.com

PhaseBio Pharmaceuticals
phasebio.com

PhysioLogic Devices
physiologicdevices.com

Rhythm Pharmaceuticals
rhythmtx.com

Roche
roche.com

Sanofi
sanofi.us

Senseonics
senseonics.com

Sernova Corp
sernova.com

Takeda Pharmaceuticals
takeda.us

Theracos
theracos.com

Thermalin
thermalin.com

Tolerion
tolerioninc.com

Transdermal Specialties
transdermal specialties.com

ViaCyte
viacyte.com

XBiotech
xbiotech.com

XOMA
xoma.com

Zealand Pharma
zealandpharma.com

Glossary

Acetone: A type of ketone body that is a simple carbon compound. In diabetes, when there is not enough insulin to get glucose into cells, the body will break down fats for energy and produce acetone and other ketones.

Acidosis: A condition in which there is an overabundance of acid. It can be caused by a buildup of ketones in poorly controlled type 1 diabetes (T1D).

Adrenergic system: A nervous system using adrenaline and noradrenaline as neurotransmitters to generate the "fight or flight" response.

Autoimmune disease: A condition in which the body's own immune system targets healthy cells in the body by mistake. In T1D, the body attacks the pancreatic cells that produce insulin. Autoimmune is also present in some cases of type 2 diabetes (T2D).

Basal rate: A rate that is set in an insulin pump to deliver insulin to maintain stable blood glucose.

Blood glucose levels: A target that diabetes patients and their healthcare team try to manage. Blood glucose levels vary during the day, and this varies from person to person. Less than 100 mg/dL after fasting (not eating) for at least eight hours or less than 140 mg/dL two hours after eating are considered normal blood glucose levels.

Blood lipids: Fat-like substances in the blood. The body needs small amounts of lipids to function normally. An excess of blood lipids can deposit on your blood vessel walls, which will increase your risk of heart disease.

Cardiologist: A physician with special training in finding and treating diseases of the heart and blood vessels.

Cardiovascular disease: Heart and blood vessel disease, also called heart disease.

Celiac disease: An inheritable autoimmune disorder. People with celiac disease should follow a strict gluten-free diet, because when they ingest gluten, their immune system attacks/damages the small intestine, which results in poor nutrient absorption.

Circadian rhythm: Physical, mental, and behavioral changes that follow a roughly 24-hour cycle. It is generated by the body itself but can be modified by light and temperature and other environmental factors.

Endocrinologist: A physician trained to diagnose diseases related to those glands that release hormones.

Epidemiologist: A public health professional who studies the patterns and causes of diseases or other health problems in order to treat the current disease and prevent future outbreaks.

Etiology: The science dealing with causes of a disease.

Glucagon: A hormone produced by alpha cells in the pancreas. In response to low blood glucose levels, glucagon is released to regulate the utilization of glucose and fats. Thus, glucagon keeps blood glucose levels high enough so the body functions well.

Glucose: A simple sugar and major source of energy for most cells of the body.

Gluten: A protein found in wheat, rye, and barley.

Glycosylation: The linkage with glycosyl groups, which can happen between D-glucose and the hemoglobin chain. The level of glycosylated hemoglobin corresponds with the raised blood D-glucose level in patients with poorly or uncontrolled diabetes.

Hyperglycemia: A condition with excess blood glucose often associated with diabetes.

Hyperglycemic coma: Unconsciousness from a combination of a severely increased blood sugar level, dehydration and shock, and exhausation.

Hypoglycemia: A condition with low blood glucose that can occur in patients treated with either insulin or treatments that increase insulin production.

Hypothermia: A condition of abnormally low body temperature that is a frequent sign of severe hypoglycemia in diabetes patients.

Insulin: An important hormone made by pancreas beta cells that keeps blood glucose from getting too high (hyperglycemia) or too low (hypoglycemia). Insulin helps the body use glucose from food for energy or to store glucose for future use. In people with T1D, the pancreas makes little or no insulin. In people with T2D, the pancreas makes insulin but the bodies do not respond well to insulin.

Ketoacidosis: A serious condition that can result in a patient losing consciousness for a long period of time or even death. When there is not enough glucose for energy, the body breaks down fat for energy and produces ketones, which can build up in the blood, thus making it more acidic if the diabetes is out of control.

Ketones: Chemicals produced when the body breaks down fat for energy. Ketones can be detected by a urine test and are common in T1D.

Ketosis: A metabolic process that breaks down fat for energy and produces ketones. This can occur when there are not enough carbohydrates from food, after exercising for a long time, or during pregnancy. Thus, ketosis is a sign that not enough insulin is being used by those with uncontrolled diabetes.

Metabolic syndrome: A group of risk factors that increase your risk for heart disease and other health problems, such as diabetes and stroke. Three or more of the following five risk factors will lead to a diagnosis of metabolic syndrome: 1) a large waistline, 2) a high triglyceride level or taking medication to treat high triglycerides, 3) a low HDL cholesterol level or taking medication to treat low HDL cholesterol, 4) high blood pressure or taking medication to treat high blood pressure, 5) high fasting blood sugar or taking medication to treat high blood sugar.

Multifactorial: Involving or dependent on a number of factors or causes. Diabetes is caused by multiple factors, and therefore a multifactorial disease.

Multiple sclerosis: An unpredictable, often disabling disease of the central nervous system that disrupts the flow of information within the brain and between the brain and body. Both multiple sclerosis and T1D are considered autoimmune diseases. There are reports on co-occurrence of multiple sclerosis and T1D, while further studies are needed to determine their effects.

Nephrologist: A physician who is trained to diagnose and manage kidney disease.

Neuropathy: A term to describe nerve problems, usually in the peripheral nerves as opposed to the central nervous system of the brain and the spinal cord. Neuropathy is common in people with diabetes and the primary cause of diabetic foot problems and ulcers.

Podiatrist: A physician trained to diagnose and treat conditions of the foot, ankle, and related structures of the leg.

Retinopathy: A condition affecting the blood vessels in the light-sensitive tissue (retina) in the back of the eye. It is the most common cause of vision loss among people with diabetes.

Vasculature: The arrangement or the distribution of blood vessels in an organ or body part.

Index

Photography credits

All photography by Ria Osbourne except as stated here:

Getty Images: Caiaimage/Sam Edwards: pages 8–9; **ARNO MASSEE:** page 13;
Ian Hooton: page 15; **John Fedele:** page 17; **Caiaimage/Robert Daly:** page 19;
Westend61: page 42

Karin Hehenberger: Pages 32, 34, 40

Ryland Peters and Small: Earl Carter: pages 23 (The home of Cary Tamarkin and
Mindy Goldberg on Shelter Island) and 37 (Andrew Hoffman & Alex Bates' home on
Fire Island); **Geoff Dann:** page 46; **Dan Duchars:** pages 20 and 45; **Chris Everard:**
pages 31, 33, and 147; **Tara Fisher:** pages 24, 56, and 86; **Richard Jung:** page 95;
William Reavell: pages 51 and 54; **Toby Scott:** page 110; **Lucinda Symons:** page 103;
Kate Whitaker: pages 87, 94, and 118; **Clare Winfield:** page 111 and front cover

Tidningsmakarna/Petrus Iggström: Page 6

Acknowledgments

There are so many people I need to thank for inspiring, guiding, and helping me over the years. Without these people, I would not be where I am right now—in a position to speak openly about my own experiences with diabetes while trying to help others with similar issues. I would like to start by thanking my immediate family, including my parents, Dr Michael and Ulla Hehenberger, my sisters, Dr Lisa and Anna Hehenberger, my niece and nephew, Ingrid and Olo, and my brother-in-law, Octavio Soler. They have all been through so much because of me, but I know I can always count on them for support and encouragement.

Next, I want to thank the doctors and nurses who have been there for me when I had my transplants and also each time I have had to go to the hospital for some reason. Dr Lloyd Ratner, Dr David Cohen, and Johanna Camacho-Rivera, RN, from Columbia Presbyterian as well as Dr David Sutherland, Dr Raja Kandaswami, and Marci Siers from the University of Minnesota are the most apparent, since they were in charge of the two transplants. But there are so many others that were there when things did not look so promising. When I was crying in my hospital bed with pain or just fear, countless fabulous doctors, nurses, and technicians gave me support. Thank you!

I have been fortunate enough to have a few fantastic mentors in life, including Professor Kerstin Brismar, Jim Tanenbaum, Esq, Dr Alan Lewis, and Don Casey. They have helped me with difficult business decisions through the years, and I count them as my very close friends as well. These people do not hesitate to speak their mind, and I know their advice comes from the heart, with no ulterior motives.

I could not have embarked upon this most recent journey without my partners and supporters in Lyfebulb: Riccardo Braglia and Dr Stephen Squinto.

They are both impressive businessmen, as well as all-around good people and fabulous friends. They continue to guide me and believe in our mission.

My team at Lyfebulb has grown since my sister, Anna Hehenberger, joined as General Counsel in 2015, and Bruna Petrillo added her creative touch to the Lyfebulb brand in late 2016. I am so proud to have intelligent and good people working with me who share such an important goal: to improve the quality of life of those living with chronic disease NOW. At Lyfebulb we accomplish this by giving a voice to people living with chronic disease by empowering patient entrepreneurs and creating a strong online community.

For the recipes in this book, I would like to thank Hanna Boëthius, MyFoodMyHealth, Savor Health, Matthew Swader, and Amy Ruth Finegold (page 102), as well as, of course, Antoine Camin, Executive Chef of Orsay.

I am so lucky to have dear friends from both my childhood as well as those from throughout my career who have become very important to me. I would be remiss not to mention a few, including Mia Then, Charlotte Holgersson, and Helena Rosenblatt. All so inspiring to me, I trust them with my highs and lows, and we always have fun when we spend time together.

Finally, I want to thank a very important man in my life, Jean Denoyer. Before meeting him, my life lacked a certain "je ne sais quoi," but even more importantly, he has finally shown me what kind of woman I enjoy being. He simply makes life worth fighting for.